Return of Compassion to Health Care

V. Tellis-Nayak, PhD,
and
Mary Tellis-Nayak, RN, MSN, MPh
National Research Corporation

PAGE PUBLISHING, INC.
New York, NY

First originally published by Page Publishing, Inc. 2016

ISBN 978-1-68409-887-3 (Paperback)
ISBN 978-1-68409-888-0 (Digital)

Printed in the United States of America

Contents

Dedication

I dedicate this book to persons very special to me, three of my sisters, who taught me that the deepest satisfaction in life comes from serving others.

Louise, a medical doctor, who mended broken bodies at battle fronts in WWII, and through her retirement set up clinics in rural India. She gave me a simple advice: the best exercise for the heart is to reach down and lift people up.

Jess, a doctor of social work, spent a lifetime empowering women in India's villages. She set a high standard for me: Do something for someone who can never repay you.

Vira, a doctor of science, became a Catholic nun. Generations of college students learned from her quiet, compelling example, the recipe for happiness: If you focus on yourself, your world contracts. If you focus on others, your world expands.

—V. Tellis-Nayak

==

I dedicate this book to the nearly 5 million nurse aides, most of them frontline caregivers. I have had the privilege to work with them and to advocate their cause. Many work hard hours in trying conditions, yet serve with much dedication and compassion. They have taught me and inspired me. This dedication is but a small tribute for the joy and wisdom they have imparted to me.

—Mary Tellis-Nayak

Acknowledgements

We are grateful to the National Research Corporation for supporting this work. In particular we thank Jona Raasch, CEO of The Governance Institute, for her unstinted moral and institutional assistance from start to finish.

We are most beholden to Kathryn C. Peisert, Managing Editor at The Governance Institute. She oversaw the production with a keen eye, deft hand, and much charity.

Our coordinator at Page Publishing, Trevor Boyd, was a master at his job and a delight to work with.

Our special thanks to all those who contributed to this book in small and big ways—ideas, comments, critiques, reviews, etc.

For the record, we do appreciate those friends and family members, and especially our two grandchildren, without whose unflagging interest and active support, this book would have been completed in half the time.

Foreword

Part I
By
Kathryn C. Peisert
Managing Editor
The Governance Institute
National Research Corporation

Three years ago, my mother was diagnosed with Parkinson's disease. For most people, that day would be wrought with fear, tears, denial, anger, and a whole host of emotions weighing on the negative side of the scale. On this day, my family breathed a huge sigh of relief. This diagnosis was over two years in coming. My mother was always tall, slender, fit, and incredibly healthy. She easily fooled people into thinking she was at least 10 years younger. In the beginning of the change, we noticed my mother's movements became slower. The change was extremely subtle—not enough for most to notice except those closest to her. I recall asking her if she might have arthritis. When I asked my brother about it, he blamed it on age.

My mother had some minor chronic conditions being managed and monitored by various specialists at the time, including polymyalgia and atrial fibrillation. She was a frequent flier in the offices of her internist and cardiologist. Then she developed a tremor. Her internist thought it was a relatively common movement disorder known as essential tremor. She was prescribed medication to help reduce symptoms. She did not respond to the medication and her condition continued to decline. She began having trouble eating. She was right handed; the tremor was in her left arm. We became concerned about her ongoing ability to function independently. More and more questions were raised and left unanswered. There was never any clinical discussion about her body as a complete system; her internist focused on her shaking left arm and her cardiologist focused on her heart (he even told her at one point, "You are so much healthier than most of my other patients…"). Her providers functioned independently from one another and did not share information except at our specific request. (Indeed, this is how our current health care system is set up to operate.)

Two years and three neurologists later, with my brother accompanying my mother to her appointments to make sure the right questions were asked and answered accordingly, and a long letter from me describing in detail all of the small, minor instances of change that added up to a startling full picture, the diagnosis finally came. My brother and I had a gut feeling of what it was before it became official. In hindsight, we realized that although she was seeing excellent physicians and specialists, they were each focusing on one small piece of the puzzle. They never looked at her as a whole person. Not one asked about her ability to live her life as she desired, or compared her current movement barriers to her own, incredibly fit history. The last neurologist (her current provider) was the one who could see the complete picture.

When I was asked to assist Vivian and Mary Tellis-Nayak in preparing their manuscript for publishing, I knew this project would be a life-changing one for me. During our work, Vivian and I learned that we have something unique in common, as he battles daily with advanced Parkinson's. His passionate urgency and concern for our health care system and its reflection upon our society comes from both personal, first-hand experience and a lifetime of work researching and journaling the critical ingredients, tangible and intangible, of compassionate care.

National Research Corporation's services focus on the patient experience, using as its foundation the Picker Institute's eight dimensions of patient-centered care. This work also takes into account the experience and satisfaction of employees (including physicians), and their implications on patient outcomes. Finally, we work with health care leaders and board members in moving our care institutions towards the ideal aim of providing high quality and value-based patient-centered care. As we learn more about the effects of a patient's experience on their outcomes and overall health and wellness, health care providers and experts are building a stronger argument that patient experience and quality of care are one and the same. We are doing this work during a time of a great imbalance in American society today, as health care has been corporatized and politicized into a debate on whether health is a right or a privilege.

Human compassion is an integral component in the profession of health care. In *Return of Compassion to Health Care,* Vivian and Mary make the case that a person-centered approach requires that all care occur in a cultural climate that promotes healing. A care environment that does not take into account the needs and wellbeing of the care*givers,* in addition to the care-receivers, cannot make this vision a reality. This book chronicles the history of medicine and looks at the root-causes of how we got here today: a system in which doctors and nurses are caught in a class-like hierarchy resulting in the inability of caregivers to freely speak their minds and to work as a highly functioning team. It also results in the inability of caregivers to be fully satisfied with their work, forcing them to focus on the individual tasks at hand and not the larger aspects necessary to be a compassionate healer, which remains the original motivation and inspiration for those who have chosen to become givers of care.

This book fills a crucial gap in the literature regarding the current state of our health care system and what needs to be done to remedy it. It aims to answer three basic questions in a human-needs based conceptual framework of person-centered care: "Who is a human person? What are the primal needs of a human person? What are health care's obligations to serve these primal, universal needs?"

Vivian and Mary's years of work researching quality of care result in a culmination of stories of heroes and exemplars, across the care continuum, demonstrating that compassion in health care can and does exist. In order to accomplish and sustain it across all care settings, we need to change our perspective and focus on the human experience, for all involved in the care setting from the patient to the family to the caregivers. We need to be asking a different kind of question that goes beyond a provider's skills and experience: "As my caregiver, what can you do to make me feel whole again?" The framework in this book presents a viable roadmap for health care leaders, providers, and all of us who take part in the health care system in one way or another, to reshape the care environment and return compassion to health care.

Part II
By
Jona Raasch
Chief Executive Officer
The Governance Institute
National Research Corporation

Should health care be a universal human right? And shouldn't that care be delivered with compassion

Health care today is clearly at the center of the political debates. While there are varying opinions on how we deliver it and who has coverage, one thing everyone can agree on is that when you or your family member need access to health care, you expect to be treated with compassion. When individuals are at their most vulnerable, they not only want to receive care that is safe and error free but also want and need to be treated as if they truly matter to those who are providing their care.

Thirty years ago, Harvey and Jean Picker founded the Picker Institute in Boston. It was the first body to investigate, scientifically, not just what patients really wanted from health care but how doctors and health care providers could improve the patient experience. As Margaret E. Mahoney, President of the Commonwealth Fund at that time, said of the Pickers, "It is suggestive of their insight and sagacity that the family that quite literally built the academic base for the science of radiology should recognize an equal imperative to understand medical care from the patient's perspective." Harvey stated, "I think we are all convinced that it's possible to treat patients as human beings, meeting their wants and worries, as defined by them, and not the doctor." This journey continues, and we at National Research Corporation are committed to keeping the Picker Institute work alive and moving in order to help organizations provide, as coined by the Picker Institute in their origin, "Patient-Centered Care." The only way care can be patient-centered is for it to be delivered with compassion.

The Governance Institute works with health care boards and board members across the country who care deeply that their organizations provide compassionate care. Ensuring that their organizations have a culture that honors and exhibits compassion is an ongoing challenge. It is evident that it is important to boards. If you study almost any organization's mission you see compassion as an essential component of their reason for being. For example, the missions of the largest not-for-profit and the largest for-profit health systems in the United States read as follows (as sourced from each organization's Web site):

Ascension Health Mission: Rooted in the loving ministry of Jesus as healer, we commit ourselves to serving all persons with special attention to those who are poor and vulnerable. Our Catholic health ministry is dedicated to spiritually-centered, holistic care which sustains and improves the health of individuals and communities. We are advocates for a **compassionate** and just society through our actions and our words.

HCA Mission and Values: Above all else, we are committed to the care and improvement of human life. In recognition of this commitment, we will strive to deliver high quality, cost-effective health care in the communities we serve.

In pursuit of our mission, we believe the following value statements are essential and timeless:

- We recognize and affirm the unique and intrinsic worth of each individual.
- We treat all those we serve with **compassion** and kindness.

- We act with absolute honesty, integrity and fairness in the way we conduct our business and the way we live our lives.
- We trust our colleagues as valuable members of our health care team and pledge to treat one another with loyalty, respect, and dignity.

Vivian and Mary Tellis-Nayak very graciously provide us with an excellent framework to help us create a culture of compassion in our organizations. They share many poignant stories that grab your heart; these stories and others like them are very compelling and those in health care come away with new insights and reminders of what makes working in health care a "calling." But do we really learn from these stories and implement the necessary changes? They so rightly state that in health care, leaders, managers, and administrators are the cornerstone of sustained quality. Their passion to incarnate a person-focused vision is the best clue to how deeply an organization is wedded to humane care and caring. Every board and board member should do everything possible—in fact, it is their legacy—to create a sustaining culture that puts compassion as a solid bedrock: to be, to become, to belong, to be our best, and to reach beyond.

Introduction

Remember your humanity, and forget the rest.
—*Russell-Einstein Manifesto*

"Listen to your patient, he is telling you the diagnosis," Sir William Osler (1849–1919) used to tell his students at Johns Hopkins, where he made the bedside the lecture hall (0.01).

Osler became the regius professor of medicine at Oxford in 1905. One day, on his way to graduation ceremonies, enrobed in a striking academic gown, he stopped by the home of his colleague Ernest Mallam.

Mallam's young son lay dying with whooping cough. The child could not take his eyes off this colorful visitor. Osler examined the boy. Then he sat by the bed, peeled a peach, cut and sugared it, and fed it bit by bit to the enthralled boy. Osler returned every following day, donned in Oxford's magnificent colors, and fed the child. Within a few days, the little boy was on the road to recovery.

That was a case of health care at its best: competence and caring wrapped in compassion.

Humans are born to relate, to connect, and to bond. The most noble of human relationships is compassion, which lets us into the personal world of the other and shares the other's pain and trouble.

No other profession is as closely associated with human compassion as is health care. We rightly acclaim modern medicine's feats. It has contributed to the doubling of the human life span within one hundred years. It has successfully battled infections. It has alleviated pain and human suffering.

Although we want medicine to cure our sickness, what we as humans deeply long for is the assurance that in the trusting hands of the healer we will soon be whole again. But caring, concern and compassion are not virtues distinctive of clinical practice today. During a typical doctor-patient office visit, the doctor spends more time interacting with the computer, writing orders, and doing paperwork than in understanding and relating to the patient. Digital diagnostics have obsolesced the art of healing through sympathetic listening, the reassuring touch, the encouraging word and the kindly gesture.

The human and the humane have lost their primacy. The healing profession has grown cold and impersonal; therapeutic relationships have become an empty ritual. The clinician's preoccupation with curing the body has made the caregiver ignore the distress of mind and insecurity of the soul that illness brings. The retreat of compassion, the Institute of Medicine cautions us, has turned health care into a hazard for health in the United States. Discontent has spread among the public. Morale has slid among practitioners.

When will we see a return of compassion to health care?

This book has a modest aim. It seeks to understand the tectonic changes in health care from a person-centered perspective rooted in the best traditions of humanism. Humanism in health care places a high value on human beings, human culture, and the human experience. Illness and recovery, living and dying are part of the human experience.

Our goal is to offer an uncomplicated model that serves three purposes. First, it serves as a framework that puts in perspective and makes sense of the chaotic conditions within health care. Second, it serves as a guide that gives direction to health care reform. And third, it serves as the standard by which we assess health care's quest in the pursuit of compassion.

We deduced this blueprint from the working models of compassion in action that stalwarts have pioneered across health care. Many of them are bold efforts to reintroduce *love, caring, benevolence,* and *kindness* in every setting and at all levels. Compassion is sprouting in unexpected, even forbidding climates.

Answers to three basic questions give the theoretical direction to our framework. Who is a human person? What are the primal needs of a human person? What are health care's obligations to serve these primal, universal needs?

Mother Nature etched five basic needs into our genetic code. These primal needs define us humans; they give us our inalienable rights; they are the sine qua nons of human life. Health care's mandate is to ensure our well-being by serving these primal needs.

In a nutshell, the following are the five basic needs and rights universally shared by humans.

- The need and right *to be*
  To live, to be safe, to have access to care, and to live a decent life.
- The need and right *to become*
  To be your own self, to be free, to be in control of your life, to have self-esteem, and to be respected as a person.
- The need and right *to belong*
  To relate, to connect, to love, to be loved, and to be wanted.
- The need and right *to be your best*
  To reach your potential, to learn and grow, to self-actualize, to find purpose in life and meaning in illness.
- The need and right *to reach beyond*
  To transcend, to give, to empathize, to serve, to be compassionate.

These five drives are the common denominator of our shared humanity. Every major religious tradition has held them as sacred. They are the heart of the U.N.'s Universal Declaration of Human Rights, and the essence of the U.S. Declaration of Independence. Thus, it is just and proper that they set the benchmark by which to assess how responsive health care is to the fundamental human needs of all involved in a health care event.

In a therapeutic context, each one is a healer, and in a real sense, each one is a patient. One is lying on the operating table, awaiting heart surgery; the family is huddled in the waiting room, wracked by anxiety; the surgeon, scalpel in hand, is shaken by a bitter divorce; and the head nurse cannot erase the thought of the painful end of her mother's struggle with cancer. We are all silent patients with unmet needs; problems, personal and professional, dog us through the day. As patients, we silently crave for solace, compassion, and wholeness.

The caregivers and the support staff profoundly affect how well the patient recovers, how well the family cooperates, and how well the staff support each other. Similarly, patient engagement affects caregivers and the family. The healing of any one person depends on the contribution of all. Even the supervisors who monitor and managers who coordinate care are healers in that they ensure a proper environment in which good care and recovery occur. Unresolved troubles of one retard the speedy recovery of all. If the cure of the body requires clinical collaborative intervention, the healing of the person—body, mind and spirit—calls for a therapeutic ambiance suffused by a culture of mutual healing.

In the first part of the book, the first five chapters review medicine's past and present and set the stage for the theoretical summation of the book's central thesis in chapter 6. The second part elaborates and builds on that thesis.

Chapter 1 offers a glimpse into the content and style of the book. It presents four vignettes of compassion in action.

Chapter 2 uses the heuristic device, the ideal type, to construct three health-care scenarios that contain in live detail issues that we discuss in the book.

Chapter 3 takes a broad view of the range of health-care services and summarizes them in tabular form. We trace modern medicine's rugged early history, its early struggle to become a profession, and its ascent to the commanding position above all other competing medical systems.

Chapter 4 tracks the dark clouds that drift in at high noon. Critics noted medicine's away from its mission and the erosion of compassion. Discontent surfaced within its ranks, and distrust among the public edged toward alienation. We search for root causes and consider the burden of caregiving and the toll compassion fatigue it exacts.

Chapter 5 analyzes the impediments to compassion and traces their origins to the fault lines in the foundation of institutional medicine.

Chapter 6 presents the conceptual model that throws light on medicine's strengths and weaknesses. The model, premised on primal human needs and rights, clarifies health care's responsibility to meet the five basic yearnings of all humans. It devises a pathway for the return of compassion to health care.

Each of the chapters following builds on one of the five human needs vis-à-vis health care's responsibility and success in satisfying that need.

At the end of each chapter, under the subtitle "Models and Exemplars," we append a case study, or vignette or snippets that may not logically flow from the issues discussed in the chapter. But each of these snippets adds light, meaning, and nuance to the central argument we advance in this book.

We should note a few conventions we have followed in this book.

First, in the interest of disclosure, the two authors have worked as partners in personal and professional roles. Their professional activity has included teaching, research, mentoring, and consultation in acute and long-term care. This book draws on recent as well as past research—theirs and of others, much of it ethnographic. But it also draws on their cumulative ninety years of professional work, within the United States and abroad, and on their intimate knowledge of satisfaction survey data over thirteen years. They draw on their field notes, research, and professional experience. Unless specifically noted otherwise, every case and instance is a true depiction of what truly happened.

When the script refers to the authors, *we* refers to both the authors, and *I* refers to the one noted within parenthesis, e.g., I (VT-N).

Our discussion spans the whole health care continuum broadly divided into acute care and long-term. As we describe in chapter 2, institutional care is provided mostly by hospitals in acute care and by nursing homes in long-term care. The former serve patients, and the latter serve residents. *Medicine* sometimes refers to health care and some other times to the medical establishment. Our narrative throughout the book adheres to these and other customary classifications. But our script errs in favor of idiomatic brevity at the cost of academic purity. However, where the occasional text may seem ambiguous, the context will guide the reader to the meaning the authors intend to convey.

CHAPTER 1

The Back Drop: Vignettes in Compassion

Aim for perfection, settle for excellence.
—*Chris Mason*

We are born to relate. All through life, we connect, communicate, and share. The most sublime of human relations is compassion, a connection through which you enter the personal world of the other; you look at life from the eyes of the other, and you share the other's pain. Compassion finds its finest form in the person who gives while knowing that the recipient will give nothing in return.

Compassion lies at the heart of health care and defines its character. Compassion elevates medical science to an art, it adds a caring touch to technical cures, and it gives meaning to suffering.

But the lament is loud and clear: health care has lost its human touch; it has become too technical and impersonal.

Compassion takes the center stage in this book as we review its ebb and flow in health care. We track the socioeconomic conditions that have lately eclipsed compassion. In order to help it to regain its primacy, we lay out a strategy guided by the humanistic tradition in medicine so admirably exemplified today by stalwarts who have laid new trails laid for the return of compassion.

We jump-start our discussion with a preview of compassion in action. We present here four vignettes. We draw them from our research files. They are factual and authentic in every regard except that we have changed some names of persons in the interest of anonymity. The four accounts offer a glimpse into the content, style, and tempo of this book.

Case Study 1: Elders on a Safari

Elders on a safari? Yes, ten elders from Pine Grove Nursing Home in Powers, Michigan (1.01), are on a safari. They are in Djuma Game Reserve, a nature preserve in South Africa, whose giant watering hole draws many species of animals that stop by for a drink. As part of the safari, the elders are totally engaged, observing wildlife on an average day in this open nature's Noah's ark.

You could have seen these elders recently also in Virginia's Norfolk Botanical Garden. They were watching a pair of thirteen-year-old bald eagles engaged in remodeling their six-foot wide and four-feet deep nest, big enough to hold four chubby first graders. The majestic couple of the sky had built their nest and set up residence far from peering eyes, ninety feet up on a loblolly pine. They were oblivious that in the nearby NATO Tower, scientists had zoom-focused their high-tech cameras on them. Ten pairs of aging eyes were unabashedly peeking into the personal life of the eagles as they laid three eggs in the space of a week.

These were just two items on these elders' travel agenda.

Turning seniors into online globetrotters and avid bird-watchers is the achievement of feisty Candria Kwak. She is a certified nursing assistant (CNA) turned universal worker and labeled a Shahbaz (by the Green House folks). Pine Grove, where Candria works, is a nursing home that houses 160 elders in a building that began as a TB sanitarium in 1922. She is a caregiver to the residents; she is their friend and, lately, their travel guide.

"I knew what I could do. And I saw the opportunity to do it," Candria told us simply. She linked the computer to the TV and turned them into a live, interactive touch screen device that expanded the horizons of her aging friends. Now the elders could join the live South Africa expedition and experience nature up close, unedited, and unscripted. The elders chatted live with those on elephant backs; they instant messaged them, asked questions, made suggestions, or requested a close-up shot. They even chatted with simultaneous viewers and experts from other sites who participate in the safari.

Candria did not invent anything new; neither was her approach unusual or exotic. Enterprising as ever, she applied for and received a grant to buy a computer that came with a subscription to a web-based service called It's Never 2 Late (1.02). This technology has constructed a versatile platform with immense possibilities for enhancing the quality of life. Candria, who surfs the web deftly as if it were her backyard, came across several clever applications. She paused, she imagined, and she connected those dots. Thereby, a new reality was born.

Bears, Birds, and Bees

As a nature lover, Candria sometimes led residents outdoors, if only to sing in the rain or to frolic in the snow. This time, she opened for them a world of wondrous possibilities hidden behind the computer screen. She brought them the thrill of a live safari. She brought them to WildEarthTV.com. This network describes itself as an ecosystem of live wildlife channels and broadcasters around the globe; a South

African couple initiated it in 2007. It invites you to real and virtual wildlife safaris, adventure trips, encounters with the black bear, the best bird-watching spots, organic farming, green living, and satellite programs and more.

The site is yours to use free; in fact, it invites you to share and broadcast your gallery of nature photos. It networks with many partners worldwide, including YouTube, Facebook, Twitter, and the Norfolk Botanical Garden that let Candria's globetrotters peek into the private life of the bald eagles. It also works with the North American Bear Center in Minnesota, which has brought the elders face-to-face with a black bear hibernating in her den. And all this is live!

If bears, birds, and bees are not your cup of tea, Candria will pilot you to Ustream TV. Here, some elders seemed a bit too fond of *Deal or No Deal* or *Wheel of Fortune*, while others woke up early to make a beeline to the computer to find that the third eagle egg had hatched.

And then there is Harry Nelson, a farmer all his life. At his ripe age of eighty-five, Candria lit a spark in him. Ever since she initiated the Harry-computer bond, he has been actively e-mailing, chatting, or expanding his circle of friends on Facebook. Recently, that spark flared when Harry learned that Campbell's Soup's Barn Restoration Project would donate money to restore five decrepit U.S. barns that were voted the most deserving. Nelson was all over the web, can-vassing votes for the barn of his friend, which ended up winning the prize for the second most deserving barn.

Candria Kwak spent her first seven years as a CNA and the past three years as a Shahbaz. She takes joy in helping the elders; she told us, "They are my family. They are reason enough for me to hop out of bed in the morning." When she did the night shift, Amber, her child, was nineteen and Brandon, sixteen; they went with her to the nursing home to wash the windows and do other chores. Heather, fifteen, her youngest, blossomed under the attention the ready-made grandpas and grandmas showered on her. Christmas Day a couple of years ago, the three kids did not find it odd that after a day's work, their mother spent the night by the side of a dying elder in the place of the family stranded in a snowstorm. "Some days we are just on a pilot light, but all in all, our home is full of fun and laughter," she said. Candria, her work partner, and eight other helpers make a good team. They use the elder-friendly program It's Never 2 Late to let the elders talk to grandkids daily, visit the world's greatest museums, read one's small-town newspaper, or watch hungry little eaglets.

Case Study 2: The Spirit Descends on Emma

Can religion add quality to life in advanced age? Can it do so when dementia sets in?

The search for an answer brought me (VT-N) to the Pavilion, a large nursing home located in an older Chicago suburb that has been home to successive generations of immigrants from East Europe. Many older members among them are residents at the Pavilion.

A Jewish businessman bought the nondescript building, gave it a new face, and turned it into a skilled nursing care facility. He ran it smartly as a successful business and showed sufficient concern for residents that the Pavilion never received a citation for a grave deficiency.

He executed a master stroke in the third year. He recruited Jean Marie as his director of nursing, a gregarious, freshly minted MSN with a sunny Irish disposition. Jean Marie was a refreshing spring shower on a parched day. She befriended residents, staff, and family. Programs, protocols, and practices sprouted. A truly compassionate person-centered culture took root at the Pavilion.

Religious and Cultural Anchors

A common East European ethnic culture linked many residents at the Pavilion. Jean Marie affirmed their cultural identity; she boosted their self-worth, pride, and confidence by celebrating ethnic traditions, customs, and festivals. "Still, I was humbled," she admitted to us, "to discover a blind spot in our approach. Pavilion had not realized that religion was more than an institution. Its spirit suffused every aspect of that ethnic culture."

She went on to tell me this remarkable story.

"Catholicism is the lifeblood that courses in the cultural veins of the East European immigrant. All life's milestones and transitions are marked with Catholic symbolism and tradition. Yet not a single Catholic priest had stepped inside the Pavilion in two years, nor was a single Catholic Mass celebrated within the Pavilion walls. Instead, a woman minister in secular clothes dropped by occasionally and conducted a nondenominational service.

"So I took the lead. Working together, we planned a religious event that would resonate with the residents' experience of their younger years. We recruited a retired priest. We prepared an altar, complete with fresh flowers, beeswax candles, and the wafting aroma of burning incense.

"Ahead of the appointed hour, CNAs wheeled in the frail to join the other assembled residents, families, and staff. The make-do choir set the tone. With genuine feeling and in shaky pitch, they sang hallowed Catholic hymns and chanted familiar Gregorian verses. The priest, who looked like a pious Santa Claus, donned Mass vestments that were of a bygone pre-Vatican II age. He processed to the altar, genuflected, faced the altar with his back to the congregation, and conducted the liturgy starting in sonorous Latin. The Spirit, it seemed, was about to descend.

"A hush fell over the faithful. All turned toward Emma. At a ripe age of ninety-three, lovable Emma was severely demented and, for months, had spoken only gibberish. The congregation was aghast as the miracle unfolded before their eyes.

"Emma shot out of her wheelchair. She stood ramrod erect. She thrust her hands toward heaven and, in loud, crisp, and clear words, accompanied the priest in reciting the entire Our Father flawlessly and with not a syllable out of synch."

Meaning, Security, and Comfort

A Pentecostal moment like this hints at the promise that religion holds when you creatively graft it on to resident protocol. We found an edifying illustration in a nursing home on Chicago's north side. It served ninety Jewish elderly. Its administrator, an import from Israel, had converted a prominent section of the building into a functional synagogue. We marveled at the wide impact it made on the residents. The synagogue added a new dimension to nursing home life; it became the pivotal center for residents to meet, to pray, to study, to plan, to manage, or for camaraderie.

"Most of these oldsters were not really religious in life," the administrator told us. "But now in their twilight years, having felt intimations of mortality, they seek answers to the universal human questions about life's origins, end, purpose, and meaning. Religion and ethnicity readily provide them the road maps."

The Little Sisters of the Poor (LSP) (1.03), located northwest of Chicago, took a less studied and more spontaneous route. They simply attuned the rhythm of daily nursing home life to the Catholic heritage. This order of nuns originated in France; they serve the poor elderly on five continents. These women are the nearest thing to exemplars of organized compassion you will find anywhere.

We have observed them in three countries giving witness to dignity of life of the indigent elderly in nursing homes. Our most memorable experience occurred in Singapore. A short ride brought us to the nursing home where they ministered to the economically deprived elderly. The LSP nuns were nowhere to be found—not for miles around.

The current occupants of the premises were also Catholic nuns; they were from India, of a different stripe and with a different mission. Mother Superior filled in the historical blanks for us. "Singapore has become a prosperous state," our teacher said. "Singapore follows enlightened policies as regards the aged and looks after them well. In effect, there are no needy old people here." The LSP's life mission is to minister to poor elders. They take it seriously. So they packed their bags and went searching for not-so-green pastures.

In their Chicago area nursing home, they have created a markedly Catholic ambience. At every turn, familiar religious icons, statues, images, and signs call to the residents' mind the symbolism and metaphors that, in yesteryears, the residents had reverentially imbibed in their Catholic home, school, and parish. The feasts, fasts, rituals, and obligations of the Catholic calendar affect their daily routine and diet. The chapel takes the pride of place in the nursing home. It is the anchor and the rallying post for the community, a quiet place for private prayer and meditation.

Such ethnographic evidence, abundantly found in long-term care, and not only in Chicago, speaks of the salutary contribution religion makes in advanced age. It has stirred researchers to drill down the issue to its physiological level. What neurological effects do religion and spirituality trigger in the human brain in its normal or diseased state?

Three priests who live there as residents take turn celebrating daily Mass. On Sundays, the chapel fills to capacity for a concelebrated Mass. Families who join in the Eucharistic celebration accompany or wheel in their relative. Some do so daily. As in life so in death, religion sanctifies the final hours with sacred oils and ritual. You breathe your last surrounded by family and caregivers and comforted by the fading sound of hushed Hail Marys.

Case Study 3: Strive for Perfection, Settle for Excellence

As they drove in through the gates, the team of three state surveyors sensed that something was amiss. They parked and walked toward the front door. Their concern mounted as they noted the strange silence and the absence of any human or animal presence. Then they saw the big sign on the door: Gone Camping!

There was not a soul around except a meek young girl who greeted the surveyors with a megawatt smile. "I am the only one here," she informed them—now more annoyed than amused. "Chris took them all camping. They will be back on Monday."

That was quintessential Chris Mason.

Then in his mid-twenties, Chris Mason was administrator of this Alabama nursing home, whose 110 residents had often benefited by his unfettered imagination that saw the world not the way it is but the way it should be. In this case, it was Barry, a young resident—a quadriplegic from a sad accident—who one day confided to Chris that camping was his fondest childhood memory and what he now missed most.

Chris did the research and located a camping program friendly to the frail and disabled. He was convinced that the spirit of the law was prodding him. So he packed up his entire community and went camping. The state surveyors, however, located his whereabouts, showed up, and commenced the inspection at the campsite. Chris was right. The same spirit was at work again; they handed him a deficiency-free survey.

Chris (a friend of the two authors) is the living proof of the truth "Good quality is good business." This motto is neatly dove-tailed into his personal watch phrase: "Strive for perfection and settle for excellence."

Excellence is, indeed, its own reward; it stokes your pride and does wonders to your heart. Excellence also rewards you in tangible ways. In the best of nursing homes, residents and families become strong advocates and partners in care. The census shows a healthy share of the prized Medicare and private pay customers. Satisfied families improve their home's accounts receivables—they pay bills on time, and they loathe even the thought of suing their caregivers. Model nursing homes reach the summit by dint of their committed staff. Staff become committed to managers who genuinely care for them and give them every reason to do their best. Good managers create a safe, friendly, and fun work setting that eliminates conditions that breed staff alienation and absenteeism, inflate worker's comp claims, and discourage a sense of community where everyone looks out for one another.

From Ashes to Excellence

Chris strived hard for excellence and then savored its rewards, as was illustrated dramatically in the case of Jefferson Manor. This was an assisted living community in Dallas, Oregon, that was on its last legs and tottering. Only thirty-five residents lived in the aging building certified to serve seventy. Eighty percent of them were losing weight. Staff turnover topped 200 percent. It was hemorrhaging $20,000 a month. State surveyors cited forty-one pages of deficiencies, con-firming that Jefferson Manor was in the throes of a quality melt-down, and it was served notice of a mandatory closing.

A health-care consultant alerted Chris to the dire transfer trauma the residents faced in that small town with few long-term care choices. What happened next showed Chris Mason at his best. He conducted due diligence, pleaded with the state for a reprieve, offered a concise road map, and proposed that the state partner with him in saving Jefferson. The state agreed but demanded measurable progress in sixty days.

The rescue operations started immediately. Strict guideposts kept them in focus—always put people first, implement systems, and ensure consistency. The leader, Rebekah Gottschalk, supported by Chris and his crew, made excellence seem within reach, rallied the team, offered every help, and demanded the best from each. State surveyors showed up promptly on the sixtieth day to inspect. They found Jefferson in substantial compliance.

With that head of steam, the Jefferson train chugged confidently forward and upward. Quest for Excellence, a series of checklists used to build quality care, is a Chris Mason invention. Each completed activity is logged and check-marked, keeping the organization on track and moving in the right direction. Jefferson made a quantum leap when it opened its doors to state-of-the-art technology. It made it possible to match resident acuity to staff expertise in order to optimize staff allocation; it enabled families to track resident progress, activity, and sleep patterns; it automated medication processes and pharmacy functions; and it reduced errors, relieved staff of routine chores, assigned them greater responsibility, and generally made the workplace efficient and congenial.

The results affected every department. Resident satisfaction rose. Better informed, families became more engaged. As work became meaningful and commitment brought joy, staff stabilized, and absenteeism became rare. Except for payroll, costs fell markedly throughout Jefferson. All in all, technology served as the midwife that eased the birth of the culture of excellence at Jefferson, and it rose, phoenixlike, from the ashes and kept rising until it joined the small company of the most advanced dementia care centers in the United States. In less than a year, its asset value rose 240 percent.

Flights of Imagination

Mason's passion for person-directed quality, his faith in technology, and his sharp entrepreneurial instinct keep him ever alert to new challenges that may arise. A string of innovations bears testimony to his uncanny expertise to turn dreams into products that add quality to life.

One day, Gloria, a woman in her thirties, told Chris that she was discouraged. Despite working hard hours for long years in the nursing home, despite cutting discretionary spending and saving every spare penny, she was still far from realizing her dream of buying a house. The down payment she could afford, but her credit rating did not add up to qualify as a buyer. Chris did not see a ready solution, so he invented one.

He looked at Grace's work history—impeccable. He added up her unused days of paid leave—impressive. He factored in her per-week overtime—substantial. He blended them and distilled a credible formula. He walked over to the bank and explained to them Gloria's work ethic, that she would put in extra hours and would turn her unused paid leave into cash. He laid out his formula with the numbers all pointing in one direction: Gloria poses negligible risk; she is creditworthy. Conclusion: Gloria bought her house. And thereby was born the house-ownership program that has helped other Glorias attain their dream.

Chris has left his mark in many long-term care fields: analytic software, training for managers, support for startup entrepreneurs, forming partnerships to acquire and to turn around distressed properties, fostering neighborhood volunteer service, brain status therapy. His newest project is an imaginative mystery-shopping approach to help LTC homes to conduct institutional assessment.

With all these preoccupations, Chris Mason is not a starchy sort or someone in a big hurry. He is a bubbly personality; he expounds heartily on matters he knows and listens with curiosity and interest when you broach topics less familiar to him. He serves on his church council and has been its president. He was the head coach for Oregon Junior Baseball, and the Boy Scouts of America has honored him with an award.

By any measure, Chris Mason is an exemplar of quality and compassion.

Case Study 4: High-Tech Medicine Touched by the Spirit

An unknown virus lays Argentina-born Angelica Thieriot low; she is feeling depressed by her first experience in an American hospital. Angelica's two sons were born in an Argentine hospital where medical technology lagged, but her nurse, doctor, family, and friends all contributed to a caring environment.

The San Francisco hospital, on the other hand, was a model of efficiency. Everyone knew one's role and discharged it well. Life moved as planned. They enforced visiting hours strictly. The doctors were highly credentialed. The nurses were intently busy. But nobody seemed to smile; they walked past without pausing to exchange pleasantries. They seemed not to know how to connect. Such disengaged professional care left Angelica staring at bare walls, lonely and scared. It also made her think, and she had much time to imagine.

Upon discharge, she walked out of the hospital fired up by a novel vision of hospital care. Why could we not have a medical technology that integrated spirituality, one that was imbued with values of compassion, comfort, aesthetics, dignity, shared knowledge, and partnership? She envisioned modern medicine with a heart, a healing environment that dignified the person as it nourished the soul, cheered the heart, and mended the body. She called her idea Planetree—recalling the sycamore tree under which, 2,400 years ago, medical guru Hippocrates taught person-centered care.

A Spiritual Oasis

The Planetree concept gives primacy to the patient. In an age of impersonal medicine, it struck a deep chord. Planetree, now, is a coalition of hospitals; it offers information, education, and help to hospitals to create healing environments that facilitate patient-centered care. Since 1978, the year it all began, the Planetree concept has incarnated into an alliance of more than five hundred health care organizations committed to engage the patient as a fully informed partner in one's own medical care. Planetree has taken firm root in the United States, Canada, the Netherlands, Japan, and Brazil and in diverse health-care settings ranging from twenty-five to two-thousand-plus beds.

Planetree's credo articulates its beliefs:
We believe

- that we are human beings, caring for other human beings;
- we are all caregivers;
- caregiving is best achieved through kindness and compassion;
- safe, accessible, high-quality care is fundamental to patient-centered care;

- in a holistic approach to meeting people's needs of body, mind, and spirit;
- families, friends, and loved ones are vital to the healing process;
- access to understandable health information can empower individuals to participate in their health;
- the opportunity for individuals to make personal choices related to their care is essential;
- physical environments can enhance healing, health, and well-being; and
- illness can be a transformational experience for patients, families, and caregivers (1.04).

Griffin Hospital in Derby, Connecticut, houses Planetree's central operations (and is a Planetree affiliate). This modest, 160-bed community hospital stands likes a colossus of quality. Every connoisseur and authority, from The Joint Commission to the AARP, has heaped highest honors on it as "number one in Connecticut," "one of top ten healing hospitals in America," "among the top 5 percent for patient satisfaction and an exceptional patient experience," and "for its high degree of community value."

In our sojourn at Griffin Hospital, we lingered longer at three departments (OR, ER, and radiology) where the protocol demands heavy reliance on technology, gives maximum autonomy to the clinical experts, and leaves little room for the niceties of compassion and the nuances of person-centered care. At this Planetree site, nurses and doctors work as a well-knit community, supportive of one another, with negligible turnover, long tenure, and ever attentive to the personal needs of patient and family.

- The ER nurse attending on a homeless child, a patient, takes her to a toy store and lets her pick her favorite panda bear.
- Families visit all hours, bring food for their family member, and have easy access to their patient's chart and the physician's notes. They participate in care planning and caregiving, especially at crucial times like surgery.
- A Catholic nun follows ER patients and engages each of them in a narrative therapy.
- A compassionate nurse finds that her male patient has lost all his earthly possessions in a fire; she drives him to Target to be suited up.
- Doctors in radiology seek feedback from patients discharged after mastectomy; they learn about the discomfort the patients experience wearing the seat belt while they drive. As a follow up, they engage the patients in inventing a heart pillow to alleviate the postsurgical discomfort.
- The doctors and nurses keep close contact with patients after discharge, engage them in educational programs that teach self-management, and rely on them to learn about their postdischarge needs and how the hospital can serve them better.

Navigating the Long-Term Care Waters

Bold initiatives, it seems, are coded in Planetree's cultural DNA; Planetree has engendered not a few innovative leaders. Among these is Susan Frampton, president of Planetree (who topped the list of Tom Peters' Superstar/Top 41 Entrepreneurs). With senior director Heidi Gil by her side, and the skills she learned as a medical anthropologist, Frampton deftly steered the Planetree ship into the long-term care waters. This massive initiative found early success. Since 2003, more than one hundred continuous care communities have answered the call and now, as affiliates, proudly march to the Planetree beat.

Without pausing to savor the success, Heidi Gil was soon at the helm, again piloting the new affiliates toward long-term care's three coveted but elusive goals: achieving person-centered care, initiating cultural transformation, and pursuing an evidence-based path to excellence.

On the first leg of this journey—or phase one—Gil and her team matched Planetree's person-centric philosophy to the daily demands of long-term care. They spelled out its eleven separate dimensions in sixty-three designation criteria—the Planetree standards that are meant both to guide LTC behavior and to assess its outcomes. These criteria are arguably the most comprehensive and the most demanding in the entire arena of person-centered approaches. They affirm that care recipients are not the only beneficiaries in a person-centered environment; the staff, managers, and all other participants are beneficiaries as well. All persons share the same universal human need to be recognized, to belong, to give, to grow, and to transcend. Thus, a caregiver is no less deserving of a quality of life as is the patient or resident.

These standards are distinctive in another telling way. They aim not so much to teach the mediocre how to comply with minimum standards but they constantly remind affiliates of Planetree's lofty mission: to keep to the high road, to reach out for excellence, and to strive to add quality to life, dignity to death, zip to the spirit, and cheer to the heart.

Pathway to Compassion

An evidence-based approach to quality was the principal agenda for phase two. The team worked with onsite caregivers and converted the designation criteria into precise measures (disclosure: both authors served on this team). These measures make it possible for affiliates to track their progress toward set targets and goals vis-à-vis the Planetree mission: to benchmark their performance against the performance of peers, to identify their strengths, and to diagnose the weak links in their systems.

This high-minded agenda, now in its testing phase, is by far the most ambitious data-driven quality improvement venture ever undertaken in long-term care. Other important quality improvement ventures are currently taking place in the acute-care (hospital) setting as well.

Conclusion: A Compassionate Vision

These four cases open a window to a humanist vision of health care. That vision is wider than mere patient-centered care. A person-centered approach looks beyond effective treatments. It aims to create a compassionate healing culture that is sensitive to the unmet human needs of all the participants in a health-care setting.

Candria, in the first case, demonstrates that the human yearning to be yourselves, to be a better person, to grow in mind and in spirit is very much alive and active in old age. She connects the elders to other worlds, the world of their grandkids, the world of animals, the world of ideas. She fosters bonds that transcend distinctions of age, gender, race, and class.

Jean Marie, the DON in the second episode, displays uncanny insight into our shared human need to belong and to be part of a community. She draws on ethnic pride, religious tradition, ritual, sounds and song to evoke cherished memories, to regenerate aging neurons, and to create community. The Little Sisters of the Poor and the Jewish nursing home show us simple, unassuming ways to tap into the salutary promises of religion in old age.

In the third instance, we see a champion of quality at work. Chris Mason provides proof positive that technology need not be impersonal, cold, and alienating. His case demonstrates, as does Candria's, that technology does not necessarily have to replace compassion. With a dash of imagination, we can harness technology to improve health, to build community; technology provides proof that it is never too late to grow as a person. Chris Mason, in all his ventures, has made a business case for compassion and quality. His consistent commitment to compassion and quality has never failed to yield a harvest of inner rewards and financial success.

The last vignette is a testimony to how humans can scale the highest peaks when stirred by compassion. It mattered little that Angelica Thieriot was a woman, that she was born in a foreign land, and that she was forced to lie in a hospital bed, lonely and shaken. Compassion transformed her illness into a mission impossible: to infuse spirituality into caregiving in hospitals, the secular temples designed on the biomedical model by the high priests of medicine. She was not deterred that she might be merely tilting at the windmills of the mighty medical establishment. But her vision spoke to the yearning within all people.

She went on to erect a monument to compassion—Planetree, a dream turned into a beacon that motivates us to create healing environments that can mend broken bodies and spirits around the world.

The four narratives together affirm our model of compassionate health care. They also exemplify two significant features of excellence. First, feats of excellence are truly unique and exceptional; mediocrity wears a common face. The quality of life is a many-splendored prize;

the trails that lead to that mountaintop are countless. Candria, Jean Marie, and Chris Mason exemplify rare imagination and initiative. Second, successful models of compassion, like the Little Sisters of the Poor, the Jewish nursing home, and Planetree, show innovations in compassion strike root, thrive, and bear fruit in a caring-compatible, culturally integrated community.

CHAPTER 2

Health Care Today: Two Perspectives, Three Ideal Types

> I don't blame anybody—they're just doing what makes
> sense and we have to change what makes sense.
> —*Don Berwick, former CMS administrator*

We start our pursuit of the person-centered model with a review of health care as it functions today and of the confluence of forces that have pushed compassion into the shadows.

In the interest of brevity and simplicity, we skirt elaborate descriptions and textbook definitions. Rather, we summarize the contemporary health-care scene in the United States and highlight the concepts most relevant for our argument. Next, we construct three ideal types of health-care scenarios in the context of the daily rough and tumble reality of health care.

Part 1. The Salient Features of Modern Health Care

Health care in the United States is not a system. Much of it evolved with little regulatory oversight or rational planning. We can correctly describe the resulting hodgepodge as a functioning chaos. Academics, policy makers, and people in business have devised schematic classifications of health-care services that shed light on health care from different angles.

The two charts below schematically depict the concepts we will reference throughout the book. Figure 1 summarizes the determinants of health and types of health care services:

- Health is wellness of body, mind, emotions, and spirit.
- Five factors determine a person's health status: genetic and physiological makeup, physical and social environments, psychic and emotional reserves, intellectual meaning in life, and personal lifestyle (i.e., diet, exercise, daily routine, and temperament).

Organized health care has five types of delivery: public health, biomedical health care, mental health care, psychotherapy/counseling, and complementary alternate health care.

Figure 2 classifies conventional health care, in the middle column, as a continuum of nine most common services.

- We refer to the entire range of services as *health care* or *modern health care*.
- We refer to the *acute care* services in the top half also as *modern medicine*.
- The bottom half lists long-term care services that include subacute (postacute) care, skilled nursing care, assisted living, adult day care, and independent living.

Determinants of Health and Types of Health Care

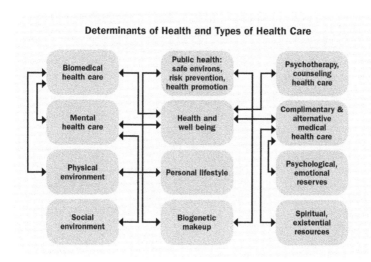

Health Care Continuum

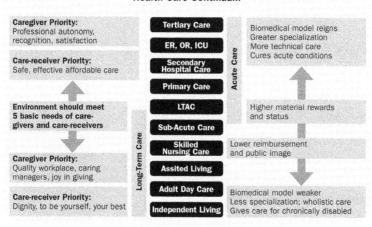

- Toward the top end of this continuum, the biomedical model influences caregiving more clearly, whereas the social model prevails toward the bottom end. Specialization, technical expertise, and clinician's autonomy are more pronounced at the top, while a holistic care, self-management, and resident autonomy play a greater role toward the bottom.

In chapters to follow, we refer to these health-care templates. We advance a humanistic, compassionate model of health care. We define a human person as driven by goals set by fundamental needs that health care has to recognize, respect, and fulfill. This person-focused approach seeks a healing environment that nurtures mutual compassion among all participants in a health-care episode (i.e., the care receiver, the family, and the caregiver team). Compassion assumes a different form and content in different contexts, as depicted in these templates.

Part 2. Three Ideal Types of Health Care Settings

What hastens or impedes the return of humanity to health care? This chapter and the following lay the ground for this investigation. In part 1, we gave a schematic summary of the elements that make up health care. In part 2, we look at health care's day-to-day operations. To that end, we rely on the time-tested heuristic tool *ideal type* well-known to sociology students (2.01).

An ideal type is a mental image of a subject we want to study. The word *ideal* does not mean you create a mental image that is "excellent," "preferable," or "desirable." Rather, an ideal type is a pure case that possesses all the features we need for our discussion minus any distracting detail. The pure image is true to life but does not exist in its pure, or ideal, form in real life. The ideal type is a didactic tool. It accentuates the aspects of the subject we study.

We construct three ideal types of care receivers in real health-care scenarios. The cases provide the living context for our discussion of compassion in this book. The three profiles are ethnographically sound, psychologically authentic, and true to life. We constructed them from the case studies in which we were participant observers. Details of behavior, feelings, thoughts, and speech in this narrative are factual and based on our field notes. Some minutiae are literary fillers and do not affect the substantive narrative.

Ideal Type 1. Harold Maxwell

Harold Maxwell, a fictional character, is our first ideal type. He is a fifty-six-year-old lifelong high school science teacher who returned home two days ago from the hospital via a rehab nursing home. This was Harold's second brush with death; the first cardiac arrest occurred twenty-two months ago. This time, an ambulance took him to the same highly regarded university-based Midwestern hospital. For the second time, he survived a complicated cardiac surgery; he spent eight days in the hospital bed. Then they transferred him to a nursing home. After twenty days, the nursing home coordinated his return home.

Last night, Harold slept well till a nightmarish dream shook him awake. The numbers he had read yesterday played in his mind. *How lucky of me,* he thought. Nine hundred thousand people in the United States suffer acute myocardial infarction each year. One in five die before reaching the hospital, and almost one in three die within thirty days (2.02). He had survived. He whispered a silent, sincere "Thank you" to all who had expertly pulled him from the jaws of death.

Harold's wife, Collette, went through some hassle at the hospital before they gave her a reclining La-Z-Boy chair to spend the nights with him. Harold and Collette's memories of his hospital stay are sweet and sour. They were in a teaching hospital, so clinicians of every stripe trooped in and out, day and night, without notice, sometimes disturbing their sleep or intruding on their privacy.

The doctors' demeanor bespoke self-confidence and silently reassured Harold that he was in good hands. Most were solicitous, but none seemed curious about his personal history or about the woman by the bedside and her role. Mostly, they went to his bedside unprepared. They had obviously not consulted with the experts who had visited earlier; their explanations and advice did not always match. At the bedside, they scrolled up and down on the tablets even as they directed some questions toward him. They addressed one another as Doctor or Mister or Miss, but they invariably addressed him as Harold.

Younger men and women followed some doctors, exaggeratedly attentive to and hanging on every word of clinical jargon of the leader. They were focused on their work and remarkably uncurious about his biography. They seemed always eager to move on, so Harold did not impose on their time with questions that nagged him. Harold and his wife observed both doctors and nurses discussing Harold's case, often out of earshot but not always; it puzzled him why they could not share some information with him.

Harold knew quite a bit about nonconventional therapeutics through a colleague at work who read everything about healthy, holistic living. Harold had anticipated that a university-based hospital would offer complementary therapeutics—hopefully, at least a massage. He felt hurt when he inquired and the nurse laughed. He was doubly sore when they did not allow his parish priest, also his spiritual father, to visit; he had come outside of visiting hours.

Yesterday's mail brought Harold belated self-care instructions from the hospital. He could not believe his eyes. The detailed instructions they sent him were meant for a patient returning home after a kidney transplant! His wife called the hospital; she was puzzled that the person at the hospital did not seem surprised and offered only a perfunctory apology.

That glaring lapse brought to mind what Harold did not want to think about. He recalled that he lay there in the post-op recovery room, alone, when panic gripped him as he remembered what happened to him in this very room two years ago. An orderly had wheeled him into this recovery room. And they left him there alone for eight frightful hours.

And that nightmare came with a bill. When the bill came after his first heart attack, Harold wondered how much it cost to get sick in America. He stumbled onto some curious facts. An average American is less than poorly informed about health-care costs in general and hospital costs in particular. User-friendliness is the first commandment in the consumer age; still, hospital billing statements can be intimidating. Harold found that the average total cost of a severe heart attack, including direct and indirect costs, is about $1 million. Direct costs include charges for hospitals, doctors, and prescription drugs, while the indirect costs include lost productivity and time away from work. The average cost of a less severe heart attack is about $760,000. Of the $2.7 trillion health care spending in America in 2011, 31 percent was spent on hospital services, i.e., it averaged $3,949 per day and $15,734 per stay (2.03).

Heart Breakers

- The Monday and Tuesday after moving the clocks ahead one hour in March is associated with a 10 percent increase in heart attacks. This risk decreases by about 10 percent when falling back in October.
- People who live alone are twice as likely to have a heart attack or sudden cardiac death as those who live with a partner or roommate.
- A person is more likely to have a heart attack on Monday morning than on any other day of the week.
- The British Medical Journal published a study that concluded that having an orgasm at least three times a week cuts men's risk of death due to heart disease by half.
- Laughter relaxes and expands blood vessels. Negative emotions lead to heart attack and stroke; happier people are less at risk.
- Moderate drinkers have 20-40 percent less coronary heart disease than non-drinkers.
- Heart attack deaths are highest in Mississippi and lowest in Minnesota.

It appeared to Harold the system was set up to shield both patients and doctors from knowing the precise cost of a procedure. First, hospital costs vary depending on where a hospital is situated and who winds up paying the bill—the patient, an insurance company, or a government program like Medicare or Medicaid. Coronary artery bypass surgery costs less than $10,000 in Argentina, $16,500 in Germany, and $67,500 in the United States. Within the United States, costs for a procedure can vary over 400 percent within a county and even within the same city (2.04). In general, of the total direct cost, hospital expenses add up to 60 to 80 percent, physician payments to 13 to 19 percent and post-acute care 7 to 27 percent.

Second, it occurred to Harold that there may be a latent function to all this obfuscation about health-care costs. A patient is offered options and what cost she or he may directly incur. But neither the doctor nor the patient thinks that an individual's rational choice may indeed be an unreasonable drain of our collective resources. We rush to get on board because the price is right, but we are unaware that we are straining the carrying capacity of a sinking Titanic.

Overall, Harold thought, the nurses and aides were much nicer than the doctors—especially the CNA Vanessa, who connected with Harold the person hiding behind Harold the patient. She was solicitous, her voice had a joyous tilt, and she was never rushed. She shared her personal stories and seemed eager to listen to Harold's. Nurse Aiysha was something else. She stood ramrod straight, and she was efficient and competent; she answered him in sounds, not words. Most RNs were personable; many were kind, although not all were obviously competent. As science teachers, Harold and his wife were shaken a bit, observing doctors and nurses taking shortcuts in matters of safety and infection, especially when they thought nobody watched.

The nursing home life, which Harold had anticipated with some dread, turned out to be more congenial than the hospital. Here, staff and residents smiled, laughed, and joked family style. The decor was nothing to brag about; the furnishings and equipment were tired looking. It took Harold a week to get his mind aligned to his heart. Then he let go and began to savor his stay.

The Maxwells were grateful that Harold had beaten the odds and survived. The war was not over. Harold had more battles ahead.

As other modern afflictions do, this malady did not merely target the body; it mounted an assault on Harold the person. It defeated Harold's body and had him prone and prostrate. It robbed his self-confidence and dealt a blow to his self-esteem; it planted dread prognoses in his imagination; anxiety wracked him through sleepless nights and fear-filled days. With no clue as to their cause, purpose, or fallout, fear and frustration led Harold to the edge of melancholia.

Harold also bore the brunt when his adversity inflicted collateral damage. It strained and put to the test his relations with his family, his friends, his boss, and his church. No surprise, it even threatened to make him penniless and destitute.

At long last, Harold was at the end of the tunnel. Finally, he was ready to go out in daylight and set to go home. That was when reality dealt another blow. His victory, the doctor told him, was only a truce; his infirmity would stalk him for life. Its scars on body and mind would stay on as unkind reminders of his loss. Anxiety would keep him tossing through the night, looking for answers to questions with no answers. "Am I out of the woods?" "How will I clear the mountain of bills that keep coming?" "What will it take to patch together my social network, now in tatters?" "How long will my fellow teachers pitch in for me with a smile still on their face?" "Will it be the last straw if I again request the principal for special treatment?"

Harold and his family were on their own, fighting their private demons.

Ideal Type 2. Diane Schneider

Diane Schneider is the second ideal type, a composite constructed out of our ethnographic data. Diane, a woman on the mature side of forties, finally arranged to visit the doctor. Diane had an abdominal pain and a loss of blood for three weeks. But she postponed seeking medical advice because the pain had not been intolerable; she was also afraid that the doctor would confirm her worst fears. But family and friends offered both advice and diagnosis, free of charge.

She was sitting just outside the doctor's office, agitated, anxious, and ready to grasp at any straw of hope. An unsmiling nurse dropped in, took her vitals, and quickly read the symptoms Diane described on the sheet. Diane could not resist reaching out for the straw; she asked the nurse how she interpreted Diane's symptoms. The nurse responded predictably: "I am not free to say. The doctor will talk to you about it." That answer, its flat tone, and the nurse's affect made their mark—Diane's blood pressure spiked.

Dr. Murphy, with a bearing of age, authority, and experience, showed up seventeen minutes late, which did no good for the patient's blood pressure either. He was barely finished with his questions when Diane launched her earnest narrative. She told the doctor more about her fears and the stress of family life than about her abdominal pain—what he was interested in. The doctor learned nothing useful after the first minute of the monologue. He had heard that story repeated as earnestly a hundred times; he knew its twists and turns as well as its ending. So he tried to be efficient; he turned his eyes, unobtrusively, he thought, from the long-winded patient to the computer as his mind summed up what he was about to record. He resisted Diane's bait to engage in small talk.

Miscommunication did its mischief. This office visit was heading for a crash. An emotional firewall now stood between doctor and patient. For sure, the doctor did not give Diane 100 percent attention; paperwork and the previous hypochondriac patient detained him a bit too long. He was running late and needed to be efficient if he had to meet his expected patient load. He could not spare any time for chitchat.

Despite Dr. Murphy's good intentions and gentlemanly ways, the communication went awry. Dr. Murphy was speaking to Diane in two languages simultaneously. His body language was telling Diane something very different from what his words were saying. It was telling her that the doctor, in truth, did not take her seriously. He had no patience to listen, no appreciation for how she felt; he thought her problem was located not so much in her abdomen as in her head. Diane felt betrayed. She was angry. She could feel the pain sneaking into her stomach, but she did not make the follow-up visit Dr. Murphy suggested.

Then Diane bravely called Dr. Louise McNichols. Jeri, a colleague at work, had spoken glowingly about her and had given the doctor's card to Diane. Diane had kept it because of its fanciful design.

The rush and hurry that she had expected were not what Diane saw as she walked through a mini rose garden in blossom; she stepped into an environment that was qualitatively different from Dr. Murphy's office, both in what it included and what it lacked. The fresh flowers in the garden and the arrangements inside; bright, harsh lights replaced with subdued, thoughtful lighting; wall decor that did not flaunt credentials and awards nor presumed to teach through medical graphics and pictures of body parts; the furniture was not overbearing or elitist but homey and comfortable—this was not a setting for an office visit; it was an invitation to relax, to relate, and to reach out.

The first thing Diane sensed was the faint, delicate fragrance of lilac (no doubt from the essential oils and fragrances common to holistic medicine). Diane's nerves silently assured her that she had come to the right place. Here, there were no symbols or social rituals of hierarchy. Differences had not become inequality. No gatekeeper, nurse, or receptionist guarded access to the doctor. Dr. McNichols ("Call me Louise") was right there; she greeted Diane with a hug and "Diane! Where are Kevin and Shirl? Your kids? I thought you would bring them along." Diane felt the subtle reassurance in the extra second Louise prolonged the hug. She had never met Louise before; she only spoke to her on the phone for ten minutes last week; the doctor's solicitude touched her.

The two sat at a small roundtable. The doctor did not talk to Diane; she dialogued with her, and she related to her. Expertly she guided Diane through her health history, helping her identify incongruities and stress points. Diane began to realize that she needed to change her ways and spare herself and her family the serious consequences if she did not act soon. They connected with each other as humans. Their dialogue included the joy and peril of mothering teenagers; they exchanged tips and gave advice.

The doctor instructed her on diet, relaxation, and prayer. "I will sum up our findings and the regimen we have agreed upon," Louise told Diane. "You will find my notes on our secure website. Please read, add your thoughts. We will adjust our plan as we move forward." She also gave Diane two complimentary vials of essential oils known to bring deep sleep. Diane felt they were a team and, together, would get the better of the ulcerative colitis.

"Call me in two days, Thursday, and let me hear how you are doing," said Dr. McNichols.

"Sorry, I have an appointment at the MC Bank in the morning," replied Diane.

"Really? At the MC Bank?" asked the doctor. It turned out both had an errand at the bank, so at the doctor's suggestion, they arranged an "office visit" at the bank.

On the way home, Diane stopped by the florist. She could not wait to say "Thank you" to Jeri for referring Dr. McNichols to her. This visit was a notable success: it facilitated a thorough diagnosis, it yielded an in-depth health history, it helped plan a convenient follow-up, and it ensured ongoing communication and continuity of care. Importantly, it initiated a healing within Diane; it relieved her anxiety and brought her the gift of restful sleep. Dr. McNichols felt rewarded knowing that she brought happiness and a healthy future in yet another person. She sent Diane warm thanks—Diane's tip on how to handle her teenage son worked!

Ideal Type 3. Marge Donovan

Marge Donovan, our final ideal construct, did not know that when she came to St. Pat's Rehabilitation Center, she would not return to her condo on Chicago's south side. Fast approaching ninety and a widow, Marge's condo had been home for twelve years.

For five years or more, her son, John, and her daughter, Manny, both successful professionals, watched with concern as infirmities of old age increasingly weighed on their mother. They tapped every service and resource to enable her to live in her own home. They made sure she continued, on occasion, to set an elegant, simple table for family and friends. They thoughtfully surrounded her with symbols and cues of independence, individuality, and autonomy. Her exquisite china was on subtle display, although unused since she hosted the last of her famed dinner parties four or more years ago. Her Bellaire, in spick and span condition, has kept a lonely vigil for five years, waiting for Ms. Daisy.

John and Manny came to an agreement that it was no longer prudent for Marge to live alone, given her failing eyes and difficult hearing, with John living in God's country far north and Manny a busy executive in Oklahoma.

But they knew better than to broach a nursing home as a solution. Their mother had played hysterics when they recently sneaked that topic into the conversation.

So they devised a strategy. Marge had to undergo a colon surgery. The hospital would not permit her to return directly home. St. Pat's Rehabilitation Center seemed a godsend.

Marge Donovan was nothing if not uncommonly shrewd and sharp as a whip. She could smell a wile a mile away. Not long after being admitted as a short-stay, convalescing resident, Marge figured out that St. Pat's was not a way station. Marge had arrived at the terminal. She knew why. She also knew that a protest would hardly change anything.

Still, she had to resist the assault on her self-identity. Her bruised ego needed soothing. She needed a cover to hide her insecurity and a facade of control.

So she put up a fight. She refused to eat in the dining room with the "disabled," as she referred to the residents; she ate alone in her room. She kept away from social activity but never missed daily Mass—she had no quarrel with God. She was not fully cooperative when getting a bath or when dressing. Her protest did not extend to food and eating—she had a healthy appetite. Her bouts of silence, periods of brooding, tossing in bed, frequent need to use the bathroom, and other ruses sent a clear message: Marge Donovan was pissed; they had left her in the company of ancient, decrepit biddies.

The staff was familiar with these nonverbal skirmishes common after admission. They would not be provoked; they were empathetic and took it all in stride. Marge's resistance found its mark on the family. They felt pangs of guilt, but only as deep as Marge intended. They did not withdraw empathy and affection, just as Marge wished.

Then, exactly three weeks into her stay, on the Monday of the fourth week, Marge called for unilateral ceasefire! Marge got up feisty, greeted everyone with a warm hello, and went to the board to see the activities scheduled for the day. Back on its rails, St. Pat's chugged along with an unusually happy camper who blended in with no fuss. Marge never referred to her protest or to her peace initiative. (For the record, Marge had prayed an extra minute in the chapel, had gone to confession, and received holy Eucharist the evening before.)

Marge's epiphany led her to a correct conclusion. St. Pat's was not bad! The residents were not that strange and almost like her. Most were friendly; only two women were real shrews. Two men residents were delicious company, especially when she wore pink, which soon became her favorite color.

The food at St. Pat's was nothing to write home about. It was sufficient and varied; the festive air in the dining room made it appetizing and enjoyable.

The nurses seemed to care. The CNAs were good (except Lucy, who seemed to live in the sky). The CNAs did not mind Marge's giving them tips on social grace and manners.

Lefia was by far the best CNA. She was a beauty, born in Ghana twenty-nine years ago. Lefia found time to chitchat and to give a backrub. She had mischievous eyes and the gift of the gab. She shocked Marge with her tall tales about living alongside elephants, giraffes, and mamba cobras. Marge loved the backrubs; she became friends with Lefia and was all ears for another of Lefia's African adventures.

Marge came around to refer to St. Pat's with a touch of pride as "my place." In private conversation, she still referred to racial groups using antediluvian labels learned as a child. But she proudly proclaimed to the world that Lefia was her very good friend. John and Manny can tell you in vivid detail every yarn and adventure with which Lefia regaled their mother.

The three ideal types incarnate the health-care experience of Americans in three settings—the doctor visit, the hospital stay, and the nursing home short stay. They prefigure the major themes that we amplify in the book: extraordinary cures alongside fragmented care, high clinical competence amid serious lapses in communication, technological breakthroughs and relationships lacking in warmth and kindness. In other words, these ideal types presage the central concern that an impersonal, hierarchical culture pervades health care and underlies its malaise.

CHAPTER 3

Health Care and the Biomedical Model

At medicine's high noon, the sky turns gray.

Medical sociologists call the period from the 1930s to the 1960s the golden age of medicine (3.01). Medicine was the most admired and envied profession. It wielded power over health-care policy. Its biomedical paradigm dominated and shaped much health-related discourse. By the mid-1970s, however, medicine was losing some of its luster and public esteem. Today, health care has turned too technical, cold, and less human.

We will browse through medicine's rugged history. We will trace its ascent to exalted heights, its loss of altitude, and its landing in a sorry situation, where its clientele are disillusioned, and alienation prevails in its own ranks. We will note the dire clinical outcomes that make a travesty of health care's first principle, "First, do no harm." In the following chapters, we will look for the factors that led health care into troubled waters.

Part 1. Regular and Irregular Medicine

Colonial America was hard on human health and even harder on the medical profession. As in health so in sickness, the family was the mainstay for most Americans. Through the seventeenth and eighteenth centuries, the family provided much of the care. Physicians practiced symptomatic treatment heavily dependent on bloodletting and blistering; they administrated massive doses of mercury, antimony, and other minerals as purgatives and emetics. They prescribed arsenical drugs against bacterial or parasitic infections. Fowler's solution (1 percent potassium arsenate) was a commonly prescribed tonic; in popular lore, Charles Darwin is said to have self-medicated with it (3.02).

These nostrums and treatments harmed or killed many patients, and thus, the allopathic approach came to be known as heroic medicine. For years, Abraham Lincoln took a common medicine called blue mass, which contained significant amounts of mercury (3.03).

Mercury vapors caused mad hatter disease. Many who returned to Europe in the 1800s from the United States noted the poor health of Americans, especially in the cities: crooked jaws, teeth missing, a gray pallor, a lazy gate (3.04). Historians have speculated whether mercury poisoning from regular medicine could have been a cause.

No effective laws regulated self-treatment or the making and selling of medicine, or even owning and running medical schools. Lay healers competed with physicians. Health movements flourished. Doctors referred to themselves as *regulars* and dubbed rival practitioners as *irregulars*. Homeopathy was born in Germany and came to the United States in 1825 and struck easy root. Native American doctors, herbalists, eclectics, and Thomsonians preached botanic cures. Some preached the virtues of steam baths. Grahamites, who gave the world the Graham cracker, preached vegetarianism (3.05).

Physio-medicalists, naturopaths, and others carved out their specific niches.

Midwives were almost all women, mostly unschooled and untrained; they played an important role in health care. They did more than just help deliver babies. They practiced medicine that families had passed down through the generations. Immigrant women who learned their trade in their country of origin passed down their knowledge and skills to younger of midwives. Slave women brought from West Africa also brought with them folklore, traditions, and practices that they passed on to new midwives and mothers. Most plantations had their own women who attended births of both slave women and slave masters' wives alike and cared for their babies and children.

The Revolutionary War turned out to be a boon to midwifery. As the military conscripted doctors, midwives stepped into their shoes and provided all services the physician offered. The end of the war and the coming of independence curtailed their practice. But during the 1812 to 1815 Anglo-American war, in which the British set fire to the White House and the U.S. Capitol, their services were again required throughout the nation. Nursing during this period, for the most part, was a male vocation (3.06).

A health-care practitioner's success depended on the confidence the healer could inspire and hardly on her or his formal credentials. During the cholera epidemics of the 1830s and 1840s, the homeopaths claimed better outcomes.

The regulars faced a challenge; they had to fend off competition and win public trust. Their first move was to band together as societies that worked toward standardizing their training and fighting quackery in the political arena. The New Jersey Medical Society, chartered July 23, 1766, was the first organization of medical professionals in the colonies. Medical societies formed in other states. They and other private interests ran *proprietary* medical colleges.

Typically, proprietary medical colleges adopted an easier schedule. They eliminated a long general education and a long full-time lecture term that were required in the university-affiliated medical schools. This made it easier for non-whites and women to enter the profession. Medical schools of the day were mostly diploma mills, some peddling mail-order diplomas (3.07).

It was common for a small faculty of eight or ten to operate a medical school for profit and to split the income. There were no admission requirements, and if one faculty refused, there was always another who would offer you entry. Courses hardly included lab or clinical work; they were merely lectures, didactics, textbook reading, and memorization. Students earned medical degrees in two sixteen-week terms.

Frustrated by the increasing incursions of the irregulars, especially the homeopaths, the regulars called for a national convention. On May 5, 1847, two hundred delegates representing forty medical societies and twenty-eight colleges from twenty-two states and the District of Columbia met in the hall of the Academy of Natural Sciences of Philadelphia, Pennsylvania, to form the American Medical Association (AMA).

The AMA established the Council on Medical Education in 1904. In 1908, the Council on Medical Education asked the Carnegie Foundation for the Advancement of Teaching to survey American medical education. The Carnegie Foundation chose Abraham Flexner. Flexner held a bachelor of arts degree and was not a physician or a scientist, but he was an avid educator and operated a school. More than any other single person, Flexner shaped and designed the template for the education of the modem physician.

A footnote: Abraham Flexner arranged for Albert Einstein's immigration to the United States and his appointment in 1933 to Princeton University's Institute for Advanced Studies, which Flexner headed.

Abraham Flexner and the Rebirth of Medicine

Flexner presided over medicine's rebirth: a treatment modality transformed itself into scientific medicine. He brokered the grand alliance of medical education and medical practice with the emerging new star of science. That partnership begot the mighty biomedical paradigm that helped launch the golden age of medicine. Flexner played a dual role in this historic transformation of a key profession. First, backed by the Carnegie Foundation, he studied the medical schools of the United States and Canada and shocked the nation with a scathing report on his dire findings. Second, he channeled millions of dollars from the Rockefeller Foundation to help implement the radical and expensive reforms he had recommended in the *Flexner Report*.

Flexner's Fulminations

The *Flexner Report* refers to U.S. medical schools in 1910 in harsh words. It describes them as:

- "Wretched" 20 times
- "Utterly wretched" nine times
- "thoroughly wretched" six times
- "Hopeless" 18 times
- With no "redeeming features" four times
- "A disgrace" four times
- "Poor" 84 times

It consistently refers to the alternative systems as "medical sectarians." Finally, it finds that "the city of Chicago, in respect to medical education, is the plague spot of the country."

His blunt phraseology gave notoriety to Flexner's harsh assessment of American medical schools. He described some schools as "a disgrace to the State whose laws permit its existence… indescribably foul," and "the city of Chicago is, in respect to medical education, the plague spot of the country." He found that only 6 of the 155 medical schools met his high standards: Case Western Reserve, Michigan, Wake Forest, McGill, University of Toronto, and Johns Hopkins. He held up Johns Hopkins as the model and recommended that the profession should close all 155 medical schools except 31 if they would not or could not comply.

Flexner described what he found: "Wherever and whenever the roster of untitled practitioners rose above half a dozen, a medical school was likely at any moment to be precipitated. Nothing was essential but professors.

"Little or no investment was therefore involved. A hall could be cheaply rented, and rude benches were inexpensive. Janitor service was unknown and is even now relatively rare… The schools were essentially private ventures, money-making in spirit and object. A school that began in October would graduate a class the next spring; it mattered not that the course of study was two or three years… Income was simply divided among the lecturers, who reaped a rich harvest, besides, through the consultations which the loyalty of their former students threw into their hands" (3.08).

And Flexner bemoaned, "For 25 years past there has been an enormous over-production of uneducated and ill trained medical practitioners. This has been in absolute disregard of the public welfare and without any serious thought of the interests of the public."

Flexner found no medical sectarian schools in Canada. He found thirty-two in the United States: fifteen homeopathic, eight eclectic, one physio-medical, and eight osteopathic. He assessed each by the lofty standards and the lofty outcomes that he expected of every school (i.e., training that creates an open mind free of preconception and dogma and follows the dictates of objective evidence, wherever it may lead). By this yardstick, the alternate medical systems came out so short that Flexner wondered why they should exist at all. He questioned, "Whether in this era of scientific medicine, sectarian medicine is logically defensible."

He said, "Mechanic-therapists, and several others, are not medical sectarians, though exceedingly desirous of masquerading as such; they are unconscionable quacks, whose printed advertisements are tissues of exaggeration, pretense, and misrepresentation of the most unqualifiedly mercenary character. The public prosecutor and the grand jury are the proper agencies for dealing with them."

He described homeopaths, chief rivals of physicians, with unsparing words. Of the fifteen homeopathic schools, only five demanded a high school education for entrance. Only three possessed the necessary equipment for the effective routine teaching of the basics. But they had no full-time faculty and no future.

"Six [homeopathic] schools are utterly hopeless; one is without plant or resources; the other five, are filthy and neglected… In one, no branch is properly equipped; in one room, the outfit is limited to a dirty and tattered manikin; in another, a single guinea pig awaits his fate in a cage… At another, the dean and secretary have their offices downtown; the so-called laboratories are in utter confusion.

"The eight osteopathic schools fairly reek with commercialism.

"The eclectics are drug mad… Of the eight, five eclectic schools are without exception filthy and almost bare. They have, at best, grimy little laboratories for elementary chemistry, a few microscopes, and some bottles containing discolored and unlabeled pathological material."

Flexner's report made forthright, specific recommendations:

- Reduce the number of medical schools (from 155 to 31)
- Increase the prerequisites to enter medical training

- Train physicians to practice in a scientific manner and engage medical faculty in research
- Give medical schools control of clinical instruction in hospitals
- Strengthen state regulation of medical licensure
- Affiliate medical schools to universities
- Make medical faculty full-time professors and medical students attend full-time

Flexner had anticipated resistance by a firewall of formidable egos and legitimate and vested interests. Rather than blink, Flexner needled them with the impolitic and confrontational tone of his report.

A Formidable Coalition and an Epic Victory

The result was seismic in force and scope. Between 1910 and 1935, more than half of all American medical schools merged or closed. All state medical boards adopted and enforced Flexner's recommendations. Medical schools that trained alternate practitioners like electromagnetic field therapy, phototherapy, eclectic medicine, physio-medicalism, naturopathy, and homeopathy were told either to drop these courses from their curriculum or lose their accreditation and underwriting support. All complied with the report or shut their doors (3.09).

The AMA forged an unbeatable coalition that won an epic victory. Rockefeller money, Flexner's ideas, AMA's lobbyists, prestige of science, and a like-minded FDA opened battle on many fronts: the courts, universities, state capitals, and corporate boardrooms. This coalition used tactics both fair and less worthy. It vanquished its rivals.

The AMA played a key role; it was feared for its harsh tactics. From 1860 to the early twentieth century, the AMA had a consultation clause in its code of ethics: members could not consult with a medical doctor who practiced homeopathy; they could not treat a homeopath's patients. In 1881, the AMA kicked out the Medical Society of New York because it admitted medical doctors prescribing homeopathic medicines (3.10).

The AMA's Council on Medical Education spearheaded AMA's educational agenda. Morris Fishbone headed the AMA and its *Journal of the American Medical Association* (*JAMA*) for twenty-five years (from 1924 to 1949). His dictatorial ways helped fill the AMA coffers and defeat rival medics, whom he vilified as charlatans in his speeches and editorials. He was trained as a clown, he was a mediocre medical student, he graduated from Chicago's Rush Medical School in 1912, and he never practiced medicine before coming to the AMA.

He required corporations to place expensive ads in the *JAMA*. With no drug-testing agencies around, he decided on his own that drugs could be sold to the public based on their advertising expenditures. The notorious Rife and Hozely scandal that he initiated forced him to leave the AMA. Today he is memorialized by the Morris Fishbone Center for the History of Science and Medicine that he endowed at the University of Chicago, the beneficiary of the munificence of Rockefeller who said it was "the best investment [he] ever made" (3.11).

The second partner who added financial muscle to the coalition was oil magnate J. D. Rockefeller. Educational reform helped him expand his financial influence into medical schools. JDR founded the Rockefeller Foundation in 1913, which soon focused on medical education. Simon Flexner, MD, brother to Abraham Flexner, was the first director of the Rockefeller Institute for Medical Research that later became Rockefeller University. He became a trustee of the Rockefeller Foundation.

After the *Flexner Report* was published, JDR brought Abraham over to the Rockefeller Foundation. The foundation helped turn every recommendation in the *Flexner Report* into reality. The sheer volume of the financial support deluged the opposition and washed away every hurdle along the way. Among the top grant recipients were Johns Hopkins, Harvard, Kettering, and the University of Chicago, which alone received $35 million of the Rockefeller Foundation funds. In 1928, the Rockefeller Foundation gave money to eighteen medical schools across fourteen countries.

The giant that he was among philanthropists, JDR stood even taller among businessmen. His charitable foundations frustrated what the Sherman Antitrust Act intended: to curb the monopolistic practices that had given JDR control over 84 percent of the crude oil refined in the United States. His involvement in medical education was in keeping with his investments in petrochemicals and pharmaceuticals. His donations required the recipients to comply with Flexner's stipulations and to abandon traditional, natural medicines and procedures. The medical schools' boards of directors were required to include Rockefeller employees.

Up until World War II, the Rockefeller Foundation provided more foreign aid than the U.S. government.

A curious footnote: throughout Rockefeller's adult life, he received homeopathic care. He lived to ninety-eight years of age; his homeopath died at age ninety-three.

The third partner in the victorious coalition was the FDA, more a cheering bystander than an active combatant. It began as a Division of Chemistry in the U.S. Department of Agriculture in 1883. The modern FDA came into being in 1913—the same year the Rockefeller Foundation was created. Changes in the FDA were often occasioned by tragedies that inflamed smoldering public anger and demand for effective monitoring of production of food, medicines, and accoutrements of human life. Adulteration and mislabeling of food and medications had angered the public. Urban industrial zones harbored fetid, rotten pockets. Upton Sinclair's *The Jungle*, the 1906 shocking exposé of the unsanitary and dangerous conditions in meatpacking plants, became an immediate best seller. Other appalling revelations deepened public concern about the hazards of the marketplace. FDA head Harvey Washington Wiley built alliances with groups dedicated to community improvement, like the General Federation of Women's Clubs, and advocated for government intervention. In June 1906, President Theodore Roosevelt signed the Food and Drug Act into law. The Elixir tragedy (the deaths of more than one hundred people after using a drug that was clearly unsafe in 1937) led President Franklin Delano Roosevelt to sign the new Food, Drug, and Cosmetic Act on June 24, 1938.

Its fervent opposition to irregular practitioners and its excesses in burning books put the FDA at odds with the public. For the most part, however, the FDA has worked hand-in-hand with the Rockefeller Foundation and American Medical Association and has drawn criticism for it.

Thus, the confluence of philanthropy, public welfare, and personal and professional gain assured the AMA's dominance, gave it control over medical training and practice, and aligned health care with biomedicine.

By hitching its wagon to the rising star of science, professional medicine became associated with the momentous happenings in Europe; it shared authorship of the rapid advances in biological and physical sciences and gained credit for the immense benefits medical science brought to human health and welfare. In effect, this strategic victory of the regulars in the scientific arena closed the entry into health care for its rivals.

Part 2. The Biomedical Model at High Noon

The biomedical model is the hallmark of modern medicine. The paradigm shapes how clinicians and the public think about health, illness, and cure. As an ideological road map, it guides health policy, priorities, protocols, and practices. The assumptions and logic of this theory hold a great sway; they are woven into the modern mind-set. The omnipresence of the biomedical mind-set in modern life is reflected in the simple-minded measure of the ubiquitous use of the word *clinic*, which etymologically refers to treatment at the bedside but is used in many nonclinical contexts to project an image of high standards: sports clinic, fishing clinic, auto clinic, and comedy clinic—examples drawn from our neighborhood!

The biomedical model portrays a human being as Descartes did in the first half of the1600s. René Descartes altered philosophical discourse by famously declaring, "I think. Therefore, I am." Descartes is the author of the Cartesian coordinates and was an early advocate of the evidence-based scientific approach. He argued for dualism as an effective scientific methodology to study human life: the human body works like a machine; it has material properties and runs on laws of nature. The soul (the mind) is nonmaterial and does not follow the laws of nature.

Thus, in a dualistic medical science, the human body is essentially no different from an automobile, a well-designed system of interacting parts. Good health in this context is a well-functioning machine, fine-tuned and primed to cruise through life. Ill health, it follows, is a dysfunction that occurs when some parts break down, misalign, or wear out. A medic, in this view, is a well-trained bio-scientist-engineer with the knowledge and skills to put the human machine on pause or to jump-start it and to clean, renew, or replace its parts. The biomedical thinking considers medicine as distilled science.

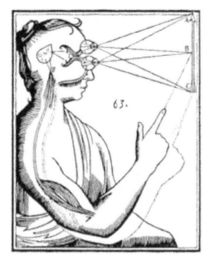

Rene Descartes' illustration of Mind-Body Dualism

Incoming information is passed on by the sensory organs to the epiphysis in the brain and from there to the non-material spirit.

Dualism as a paradigm and the biomedical model as its offshoot have held a seductive intellectual appeal, and for good reasons. Dualism proposes a conceptually elegant and convincing argument (as in the persuasive germ theory); it has been validated by its empirical outcomes—the explosion of knowledge on the biological front and by the incredible chemical and surgical interventions that have been a boon to mankind. During medicine's golden age, the biomedical philosophy ruled minds, shaped policy, and influenced every aspect of health care. Its principles and method affected life beyond the world of medicine.

The New England Journal of Medicine (*NEJM*) reviewed at the end of the millennium the most important medical developments of the past five hundred years. They chose only those developments that changed the face of clinical medicine (not preventive medicine or public health or health-care delivery or medical ethics). They presented them in eleven categories in rough chronologic order. We excerpted its salient points and present them as a table in Appendix B.

With public accolade for the blessings it showered on mankind, health care marched from glory to the very top as the most respected and handsomely rewarded of all professions. The AMA emerged as a powerful force that could hold at bay any legislative agenda it deemed unfriendly to its interests.

Part 3. Gathering Clouds: Discontent, Turmoil

Then, at high noon, the health care sky turned gray, medicine's luster wore off, and its hidden flaws came to light. A multitude of studies exposed medicine's weak links. Among the notable critics were Thomas McKeown and Gordon McLachlan (*Medical History and Medical Care: A Symposium of Perspectives*, 1971), Johaan Powles (*On the Limitations of Modern Medicine*, 1973), Rick Carlson (*The End of Medicine*, 1975), and Ivan Illich (*Medical Nemesis: The expropriation of Health*, 1976) (3.12).

Loss of Public Faith

By the mid-1970s, the euphoria of medicine's gilded age was giving way to public skepticism and discontent. Disaffection deepened in the following decades. Most surveys today show that about 2 percent of residents and families in nursing homes rate them as poor. Health care in general and hospitals in particular fare worse in the public eye. The Harvard School of Public Health, in partnership with the Robert Wood Johnson Foundation and National Public Radio, conducts ongoing surveys on health issues. Researchers studied a nationally representative sample of well and sick adult Americans in the second week of March 2012 and found the following (3.13).

Of those who got sick in the previous twelve months, about half were very satisfied with their medical care and 4 percent were very dissatisfied. Two in three said health care had serious quality problems, and one in three thought that quality of care had gotten worse. Their litany of grievance was long: 58 percent received more tests or drugs than they needed; 13 percent received the wrong diagnosis, treatment, or test; 18 percent did not get tests they needed; 15 percent were tested or treated unnecessarily; 25 percent did not receive needed information about their treatment or prescriptions; 23 percent of those seeing multiple medical professionals bemoaned that nobody kept track of the various of the treatments; 26 percent complained their condition was not well managed; 30 percent said a doctor, nurse, or practitioner did not spend enough time with them; and 75 percent wanted their doctor to spend time discussing broader health issues.

The hospital received poor grades. The report card said one in ten among those recently hospitalized were very dissatisfied with the quality of hospital care they received; one in three did not get good value for their money. Results show 11 percent received the wrong diagnosis, treatment, or test; 8 percent got an infection in the hospital; 34 percent complained that nurses were not available when needed; and 30 percent said their doctors and nurses communicated poorly among themselves. Three in five thought fraud and abuse by some hospitals, doctors, and nursing homes was a major reason for poor quality of care (3.14).

The public loss of faith is also evident in the exodus of patients to complimentary and alternate medicine (CAM). CAM is a group of diverse health-care systems, practices, and products that are not considered part of conventional medicine, including such products and practices as herbal or dietary supplements, meditation, chiropractic care, and acupuncture.

The 2007 National Health Interview Survey, a nationwide government survey, found that 38 percent of U.S. adults reported using CAM in the previous twelve months, with the highest rate (44 percent) among people aged fifty to fifty-nine (3.15). Of these, only 42 percent told their physician (MD) or osteopathic physician (DO) about their use of CAM. The 2010 AARP/NCCAM survey reported 47 percent of those fifty and older had used CAM in the past twelve months (3.16).

Herbal products or dietary supplements were the most commonly used CAM (37 percent) followed by massage therapy, chiropractic manipulation, and other bodywork (22 percent). Among users of CAM, 51 percent were women. Users educated beyond high school outnumbered their counterparts in every type of CAM users.

Tellingly, 77 percent used CAM to prevent illness or for overall wellness, and 73 percent to reduce pain or treat painful conditions.

In sum, health-care recipients are disaffected and discontented. Two in three think health care is seriously flawed; half of the population breaks with tradition and seeks healing outside modern medicine. Very notably, these people are older, better educated, and seek to maintain health and manage pain.

CAMS: Complementary and Alternative Medical Systems

Complementary and alternative therapies
Therapies not yet considered mainstream and not normally offered by conventional medical providers.

Complementary medicine
The use of CAMS with conventional medicine. Most use of CAMS by Americans is complementary.

Alternative medicine
The use of CAMS in place of conventional medicine.

Integrative medicine (also called integrated medicine)
A practice that combines conventional and CAMS treatments.

A small sampling of CAMS therapies include acupressure, acupuncture, aromatherapy, craniosacral therapy, Ayurvedic medicine, biofeedback, osteopathic medicine, homeopathy, hypnotherapy, chiropracty, reflexology, and Rolfing.

Alienation among Practitioners

The disillusionment among the public finds an echo in the loss of heart among physicians. Many physicians are discouraged, sad, and angry as they helplessly watch their beloved profession turn cold, mechanical, and impersonal. Professional pride and esteem among physicians have ebbed. Over 84 percent of physicians see their profession in retreat. In 1973, less than 15 percent of physicians had doubts they had made the correct career choice. Surveys now show that 30 to 40 percent of physicians would not be doctors if they were deciding on a career again. In a 2012 survey, more than three in four physicians were pessimistic about the future of the medical profession; two in three would have retired if they had the means (3.17). Four out of five felt they could do little to change the health-care system, and 58 percent of them would not recommend medicine as a career to their children or other young people. Over 62 percent estimated they provide $25,000 or more each year in uncompensated care.

Nurses are the anchor of health care. Across age, education, and specialty, 90 percent of nurses are satisfied with their career choice. However, they are less sanguine about their current jobs—only 73 percent are satisfied, 72 percent would encourage others to become a nurse, and 51 percent of nurses worry that their job is affecting their health. A third of them often think of resigning, and a third will not be working in their current job a year from now (3.18).

The Tragic Sequel

The perilous mix of public disaffection and caregiver disengagement is an omen that a disaster is in the making. The authoritative Institute of Medicine (IOM) says that the dreaded disaster has already befallen us. In its 1999 report, *To Err Is Human: Building a Safer Health System,* the IOM concluded that a U.S. hospital may be hazardous to your health. American hospitals had failed in their sacred pledge to the public: "Primum non nocere" (First, do no harm).

IOM reported that each year, 98,000 people die because of preventable medical errors.

Some critics alleged that the IOM report understated the disaster. Among those who thought that IOM numbers fell short of the reality was John T. James at Space Center Houston. In 2010, he used refined analytic tools and developed vastly more accurate and reliable estimates of medical mistakes (3.19).

James examined studies of adverse events (i.e., preventable harm suffered by patients). He analyzed records of over 4,200 patients hospitalized between 2002 and 2008 and found that 21 percent of the cases had serious adverse events and 1.4 percent of cases had lethal adverse events.

He extrapolated across 34 million hospitalizations in 2007 in the United States and concluded those preventable errors contribute to 215,000 deaths of hospital patients annually. That was the baseline figure derived using the tools available to him. The actual number estimated rises to 440,000 deaths from substandard care in hospitals—roughly one-sixth of all deaths that occur in the United States each year.

Specifically:

- Three percent or more of hospital patients are hurt by medical error.
- One in three hundred patients die from such mistakes.
- Twenty-four percent of people say they or a family member have been harmed by medical error.
- Ninety thousand people die of hospital-acquired infections annually.
- More than half of these may be preventable.

- Healthgrades put the number of preventable deaths at two hundred thousand annually.
- Fifty-five percent of recommended care actually gets administered.
- Two thousand dollars is the annual cost to employers per insured worker due to poor quality.

Subsequently, many researchers have offered more evidence to support and refine these conclusions.

Clinical iatrogenesis has a long history. Roman law held a doctor legally accountable for ignorance, being reckless, and bad practice. A doctor who did not properly treat a slave had to pay the price of the slave and the loss of the master's income. Citizens were free to avenge malpractice on their own (3.20).

To conclude, a three-pronged adversity challenges health care today. A distrusting public has soured doctor-patient relationships and pushed back the cause of compassion. Demoralized practitioners, their professionalism under siege, have become defensive and cautious about compassion. An uncaring health-care culture lets clients be harmed, making a travesty of health care's principle, "First, do no harm."

We explore causes of these problems in the two following chapters.

Avoidable Human Error

Lucian Leape, M.D. of Harvard University recorded an average of 178 clinical interventions patients receive in intensive care units. He recorded 99 percent successful performance and 1 percent clinical error. He noted the enormity of this error by pointing to what W. E. Deming had said. Outside of healthcare, even a 99.9 percent rate of success would be intolerably low. A 0.01% error rate would mean:

- Two jumbo jet crash landings per day at O'Hare airport
- 16,000 pieces of lost mail every hour by the U.S. Postal Service
- 32,000 bank checks deducted from the wrong bank account every hour

Part 4. Physicians' Voices: 2012

The following are excerpts from the results of the *Survey of America's Physicians: Practice Patterns and Perspectives* (3.21). They express the emotion behind the numerical responses from physicians we referred to above.

	U.S. Physician Voices Open-ended Comments in a National Survey 2012 A Sample
1.	The state of the medical profession today is a disaster. With all of the regulation and documentation required of physicians and nurses, less and less time is spent with the patients. The patients are literally dying to have their questions and concerns answered by their doctor. I believe that there is a need for a universal system to cover only the basics. This would include immunizations, catastrophic disease (cancer, trauma, etc.). Everything else should be privatized.
2.	There is a shortage of primary care physicians currently. This will be even more acutely felt if too much is asked for them to do as far as regulation is concerned. A majority of them is close to retirement and will just leave if more is expected of them that have little to do with actual patient care. The current trend to increase the regulations will push more of them into retirement.
4.	It is still a very honorable profession that takes a lot of smarts, skills, and patience to be truly good at.
5.	Quality is going to suffer because administrators run medicine, not the physicians. The administrators tell us how many patients we should see, what tests we can order, how much we will get paid. No one is looking out for the patients.

6.	I recently quit my job at a local mental health center where I served as the main geriatric psychiatrist was sick of dealing with Medicare part D plan formularies and prior authorizations, sick of being told how to practice, sick of being told I had only 15 minutes to see patients, and sick of being lumped in with "mental health" or "behavioral health" organizations where I was treated like a counselor. I am now full time in my private practice. I see anyone and everyone. Some of my patients can't pay at all. I make A LOT less money. I am quickly burning out.
7.	After years of training, it is ridiculous to be following protocols, which increase cost and do not change my care. I have lost much autonomy and feel like I'm just documenting what has occurred while I was on shift.
8.	I worry every day about taking more (yes, I said more) personal loans out just to keep my practice going. Then why am I still doing this you ask? There really is no reward for continuing to practice other than knowing in my heart that I am doing a good job and patients are benefitting.
9.	The government and insurance industry is pushing the medical profession further and further away.
10.	My life has been destroyed, and therefore my happiness, patriotism, and professionalism have all been permanently damaged.
11.	"Doctors are rich" is the false perception. No one jumps up and down to pay my $300,000 student loan. How about all the sacrifice I made? I wasn't blessed with a brilliant mind or a silver spoon. I had to work very hard, forego many sleepless nights, and see my children few times per year while away in med school and residency. Isn't all the sacrifice worth something? Shouldn't I be compensated somewhat? Yes, I am bitter.

12.	Should a "time machine" cast me back to (graduation from college) I have no idea what I would do to make a living. But, it would not be medicine.
13.	Leave us alone. There was a time when I gave 20 percent of my time to indigent patients. Now I can't afford to see anybody without being paid. There was a time when drug companies happily supplied me with free samples for my patients who could not afford their products. That too is gone. Politicians do not and cannot understand medical practice. They need to keep their noses out.

CHAPTER 4

Caring in an Uncaring Setting

Moral Persons, Immoral Systems

The last chapter described the sorry plight medicine finds itself in today. What tempted health care to drift into this unenviable situation? We seek an explanation on two levels. In this chapter, we look for an answer on the personal level of the face-to-face clinical encounter. In the next chapter, we look for the root causes in the structural defects in the medical establishment.

How we view the world and interpret life conditions our response to what life holds in store for us. Paul E. Ruskin, MD, was at the podium, guest-lecturing to a class of graduate nurses who were studying the psychological aspects of aging (4.01).

He started with the following case:

"The patient is a white female. She neither speaks nor comprehends the spoken word. Sometimes she babbles incoherently for hours on end. She is disoriented about person, place, and time. She does, however, seem to recognize her own name. I have worked with her for the past six months, but she still doesn't recognize me.

"She shows complete disregard for her physical appearance and makes no effort whatsoever to assist in her own care. She must be fed, bathed, and clothed by others. Because she is toothless, her food must be pureed. Because she is incontinent of both urine and stool, she must be changed and bathed often. Her shirt is generally soiled from almost constant drooling. She does not walk. Her sleep pattern is erratic. Often, she awakens in the middle of the night, and her screaming awakens others.

"Most of the time, she is very friendly and happy. However, several times a day, she gets quite agitated without apparent cause. Then she screams loudly until someone comes to comfort her."

He stopped. He asked the nurses seated in front of him, "How would you feel about taking care of the patient I described?" As expected, the nurses were solicitous, but they expressed their feelings honestly with words as such as *frustrated, hopeless, depressed,* and *annoyed.*

He slowly reached into his inside coat pocket as he told the class, "I enjoy taking care of her." He then passed around a snapshot of the patient: his adorable six-month-old daughter.

Why is it so much more difficult to care for a ninety-year-old patient than a six-month-old with identical symptoms? The aged patient is just as human as the child. Those at the end of life deserve the same care and attention as those who are vulnerable in infancy. Both are human beings deserving of our care and concern; both may demand equal amount of time, vigilance, and personal care.

Yet we instinctively know that the two cases are qualitatively different. Each sends a distinct message about life—its sanctity and frailty. An infant represents new life, hope, beauty, and promise. A confused senior is a reminder of the transience of human life, a foretaste of the decline, loss, and death that await us.

Rational Thinkers, Irrational Behavior

How we interpret our task shapes the joy with which we accomplish it. Humans are rational. Their behavior often is not. Symbolism drives human action. Innovation and evidence-based progress in clinical care are not always welcomed by practitioners. Even well-informed professionals display this unreasonable behavior.

In our fieldwork, we were once engaged in a deep conversation with a brain surgeon. When we broached the hot topic of the day, surgical checklists, he bristled. "I took offense when the hospital suggested the checklist protocol to me. It is demeaning to use such childish toys," he said with considerable emotion. Then, he gratuitously and half-seriously added, "Gawande, of checklist fame, is a fraud."

Health care suffers from a gap between new knowledge and putting it into practice. Very many pioneers in medicine have faced opposition and ridicule. The list includes legendary epidemiologist John Snow (1813–1858) and premier chemist and microbiologist Louis Pasteur (1822–1895) to our contemporaries Barry Marshall and Robin Warren (2005 Nobel laureates who discovered that the bacterium *Helicobacter pylori* caused peptic ulcers). Marshall said in 1998, "Everyone was against me, but I knew I was right."

Bernard Lown, MD, is a noted cardiologist and Nobel laureate, professor of cardiology emeritus at the Harvard School of Public Health, and senior physician Emeritus at the Brigham and Women's Hospital, Boston, Massachusetts. In the first part of the twentieth century, he invented the direct current defibrillator for cardiac resuscitation and the cardioverter for correcting rapid disordered heart rhythms. He showed that sudden cardiac death was reversible and those successfully resuscitated could have a near normal life expectancy. The 35 percent mortality of heart attack, Lown found, was due to rigorous bed rest. Lown encountered enormous opposition and hostility among doctors to his chair treatment (4.02).

One stellar figure among these trailblazers has risen to an iconic status by the adversity he endured in defense of progress. Nineteenth century Hungarian physician Ignaz Semmelweis knew that puerperal fever in hospital births was common and killed up to 35 percent of the mothers. As the head medical resident at the Vienna General Hospital, he observed that in ward 1 (where medical students examined expectant mothers), the mortality was three times higher than in ward 2, which was staffed by midwives. Adept in statistics, Semmelweis correctly concluded that the cause of higher mortality was that doctors came directly from performing autopsies next to ward 1 and conducted clinicals without washing hands. He did not know about the germ theory, which was decades away. He first thought the poisonous miasma played a role, but his calculations ruled it out and led him to the unwashed hands.

In April 1847, he instituted a policy of washing hands between autopsy work and the examination of patients; doctors would use a solution of chlorinated lime, calcium hypochlorite because it removed the putrid autopsy smell. The mortality in ward 1 fell from 3 percent in April to 2.2 percent in June, 1.2 percent in July to zero in the next two months. This level prevailed in the year following.

But lack of cleanliness leading to sickness was too extreme a view at that time. Not unlike the surgeon who told us that the checklist was beneath him, Semmelweis's peers were offended by the handwashing protocol. They ignored him and laughed at him. Semmelweis was dismissed from the hospital. Persistently ridiculed and harassed by the medical community in Vienna, he was forced to move to Budapest.

In ward 1, doctors went back to their old ways, and fatality rates immediately increased to their level pre-1847. Semmelweis applied his findings at St. Rochus Hospital in Budapest. The death rate in the maternity units there dropped drastically.

His contemporaries, however, rejected him; like his wife, they thought he was going mad. In 1865, at the age of forty-seven, Semmelweis was tricked into visiting an asylum; there he was strait-jacketed and committed. Fourteen days later, he was beaten to death by the guards.

Semmelweis's other famous contemporary, Florence Nightingale, achieved a similar feat some years later. She was not battling germs that, like Semmelweis, she knew nothing about. She was repulsed by the malodorous, filthy environment. The British military hospital in Constantinople sat on top of a cesspool. Patients lay in their excrement on stretchers in the hallways in the company of rodents and bugs. Nightingale wrote, "The British high command had succeeded in creating the nearest thing to hell on earth" (4.03). Ten times more soldiers died from typhoid and cholera than from injuries incurred in battle.

Armed with brushes and soap, Nightingale led her crew and scrubbed the place clean; mortality dropped from 42 percent to 2 percent.

Thus, not all deserving programs survive or enjoy a long shelf life. New ways evoke resistance, especially when they require behavior change. Directly or indirectly, patients get harmed when clinicians will not keep up with the state-of-the-art knowledge and practice.

Caring Caregivers, Unsafe Care

Health care stands as a quintessential example of high-minded individuals being opted by an amoral or immoral system. The culture of a hospital and its expectations on clinical productivity not only douse the altruistic idealism of many a new clinician, it can transform and redefine the workday world into an amoral reality. Two cases illustrate how skewed are a hospital's care systems and how badly so.

The first case, with supreme irony, involved none other than Donald Berwick, MD, a leading light in health care and President Obama's appointee as interim director of CMS. For six months, from the bedside of Anne, his wife, Berwick observed caregiving at the frontline in an elite Eastern hospital.

Berwick gave the highest praise to his wife's caregivers (4.04):

"It left me more impressed than I have ever been with the goodwill, kindness, generosity, commitment, and dignity of the people who work in health care—almost all of them. Day after day and night after night, Ann, our children, and I have been deeply touched by acts of consideration, empathy, and technical expertise that these good people—nurses, doctors, technicians, housekeepers, dieticians, volunteers, and aides of all sorts—have brought to her bedside. The kindness crosses all boundaries."

He also testified to the flagrant errors he saw with his own eyes:

"We needed safety, and yet Ann was unsafe… The errors were not rare; they were the norm… We needed consistent, reliable information… Instead, we often heard a cacophony of meaningless and sometimes contradictory conclusions. We needed respect for our privacy, personal attention, and timely care. Often we got it. But often we didn't… I was not permitted to join her for almost 90 minutes, even though she repeatedly asked that I be allowed to comfort her."

The experience radicalized Berwick and turned him into an avowed crusader of patients and person-centered care.

The second case features Robin Youngson, an anesthetist in New Zealand and founder of Hearts in Health (4.05). He observed that in a consumer age, a great many industries have become consumer friendly and have improved personal service. A conspicuous exception is health care. His analysis of the situation in New Zealand largely applies to the health-care scene in the United States.

Chloe, Youngson's eighteen-year-old daughter, was tied to a hospital bed in traction for a broken neck. Flat on her back immobilized, she was unable to see anything but the ceiling. Unable to feed or toilet herself, she lay there for three months in a hospital that failed to respond to her simple human needs. Youngson had worked in this hospital as a senior clinician and manager; he had extensive networks of influence. But no amount of pleading, persuasion, or anger overrode the systemic failure and the absence of a culture of compassion.

In general, the standard of clinical care was excellent. But that Chloe did well was a testament more to the support of family and friends. "I run workshops on humanity and compassion… In every workshop I have ever run, the participants tell me that my daughter's experience is typical of what they see every day," Youngson said.

In the following chapters, we will further develop the argument that flawed systems and processes have caused compassion to whither on the health-care vine.

The Burden of Giving Care

The most effective systems may minimize risk, but they do not eliminate risk. This is particularly true in health care. Here, the highest competence is attained by practice, by taking risks, and by trying new treatments. Consider the case of Dr. Henry Marsh, Britain's leading brain surgeon (4.06). *New York Times* reviewer Michiko Kakutani writes a forceful review ("'Do No Harm,' a Brain Surgeon Tells All") of an even more forceful book (*Do No Harm: Stories of Life, Death, and Brain Surgery*) written by Dr. Marsh.

Dr. Marsh candidly runs through a list of his "disasters" in this book—headstones in "that cemetery which the French surgeon Leriche once said all surgeons carry within themselves." A woman left almost completely paralyzed because Dr. Marsh dismissed early signs of a postsurgical infection. A patient who came through surgery on his pituitary gland just fine but suffered a debilitating stroke days later that left him "utterly without language." An eleven-year-old Ukrainian girl with a huge tumor at the base of her brain, who suffered a severe stroke after a second operation, returned home more disabled than when she had left it and died eighteen months later.

"Such stories underscore the role that bad luck and terrible mistakes can play in medicine, resulting in the dreaded word 'complications': a piece of surgical equipment can malfunction; a tumor can turn out to be stickily attached to the brain and impossible to completely remove; a poor decision (even whether to operate or not) can be made; a vein can tear and flood the brain with blood, hiding everything and leaving the surgeon to operate by 'blind reckoning, like a pilot lost in a cloud.'" A trainee doctor, supervised by a veteran like Dr. Marsh, can also botch a routine procedure: "It's one of the painful truths about neurosurgery that you only get good at doing the really difficult cases if you get lots of practice, but that means making lots of mistakes at first and leaving a trail of injured patients behind you."

Deeper the Compassion, Greater the Hurt

Caregiving puts at risk not merely the care receiver but also the giver of care. A report from Seattle in September 2011 illustrated this point (4.07). Lyn Hiatt, a twenty-four-year career critical-care nurse made the only serious medical mistake in her life: she dispensed 1.4 grams of calcium chloride instead of 140 milligrams, the correct dose, which led to a child's death. Devastated and in tears, Hiatt alerted her colleagues. And then her life unraveled. The hospital fired her; a state nursing commission investigated the case. She lost her license to practice nursing, the great love of her life, and Hiatt committed suicide at age fifty.

Every serious medical error claims at least two victims: the person hurt by the mistake and the person who has to live with the guilt. Lyn Hiatt bears no link to nurse Theresa Brown, but together they illuminate our topic (4.08). Theresa was scheduled to work a twelve-hour shift but had agreed to stay on so the floor wouldn't be short-staffed. Hospital error rates go up when nurses work more than twelve hours. But Theresa had done it before, when needed, and all had been fine.

Overworked and coping with change in orders for a child with cancer, she did not fully address a leaky intravenous tube. The patient was supposed to get two drugs, and Theresa had given only one. When she was told of the lapse, she bent over with the pain of surprise. With chemotherapy, the timing of the drugs can be crucial.

"I worried that the patient's treatment had been compromised and that she might die from her disease because of my mistake," Brown said. "I felt that I had broken a sacred bond. As nurses, keeping our patients safe is always our most important priority. If my error endangered my patient in any way, I had completely failed in the most fundamental obligation of the job. But I was lucky that my mistake ended up not having any clinical consequences.

"Amazingly, the patient knew of my mistake, but once she learned that it didn't matter in terms of the course of treatment, her only concern was for me. The patient told the doctors that I had done a good job caring for her that evening, and she didn't want me to be fired."

For all we know, doctors, nurses, and other practitioners are humans, not any different from the rest of us mortals. Passion, emotion, and desire drive them; they are considerate, kind, and caring; they are prone to pride, prejudice, anger, and sin. In short, they are a normal sample of humanity. Still, many people, especially patients in hospitals and residents in nursing homes, look upon them as demi-gods, supremely competent and learned about the body and its vulnerabilities. People perceive them as objective, unbiased in ambivalent situations, and as stoic and unflappable in trying circumstances.

We want them to be present during life's anxious and difficult moments: birth, death, accident, trauma, sickness, and pain, and to help us in matters of morality, sexuality, and dying. Thus, a doctor, nurse, or other practitioner rides a roller coaster of intense sensations, sentiments, and sensibilities, sometimes all within the span of a single day.

A mature professional welcomes a clinical challenge. When you successfully perform a difficult task, you feel a boost to your pride and satisfaction. So too when your best efforts fail to save a life, you are left with a feeling of defeat.

Dr. Rooney is angry and sad because faceless managed-care functionaries have denied a kidney transplant to Jonathan, his favorite and most deserving patient. Elizabeth, a nurse for thirty years, is traumatized with the lifeless baby cradled in her arms that she was forced to let die. Marcia, the social worker, is apprehensive preparing for an imminent session with her uncouth and belligerent new client. Dr. Ambrose, a brain surgeon, beat the odds in a complicated brain surgery and now relishes the satisfaction of bringing joy to an ever-grateful and forever-beholden family. Marianne, a nurse, cannot shed the humiliation that she made an error four years ago that nearly killed a patient; fear of making another error haunts her.

A clinician's anguish is deeper when she or he places a high value on life. The gap between what doctors wish to achieve and what they actually achieve discourages and disappoints. Too many medics start practice ill prepared to achieve a balance between what compassion urges and the responsibility to be kind to oneself, to know one's limits, and to avoid compassion fatigue. Their education taught them how to treat their clients but not how they could lead a lifestyle.

Impoverishing Medical Education

Kenneth Ludmerer in his masterful *Let Me Heal: The Opportunity to Preserve Excellence in American Medicine* reviews the history of medical training. In the 1890s, Sir William Osler, a demigod in American medicine, created at Johns Hopkins a postgraduate program that required medical graduates to live at the hospitals. Ludmerer described this residency that was widely admired and imitated.

Despite their spartan conditions, these young medics eagerly sought mentorship under learned, experienced, and wise physicians. These teachers instilled a strong moral sense leaning heavily toward altruism, they practiced medicine as a calling, and they put the patient's well-being above all else. They viewed commercialism as antithetical to teaching hospitals; they made their hospitals compete with one another to be the best, not the biggest or the most profitable.

The Osler legacy lasted through the affluent post-WWII years. But as health care claimed an ever-larger slice of an ever-enlarging national pie, regulation and reimbursement schemes (DRGs, HMOs, PPS, etc.) imposed market discipline on hospitals. In order to survive, to compete, and to get ahead, hospitals adopted market ways. Sidestepping concerns of conflict of interest, hospitals signed marketing agreements with pharmaceutical, biotech medical-devices companies. *The New England Journal of Medicine,* in 1980, raised the alarm that health care was becoming a part of a "medical-industrial complex."

This commercialization, Ludmerer writes, devastated medical residency training. Teaching lost its vaulted status. Teaching hospitals today showcase and reward medical researchers and winners of grants who add to the revenue stream. Just a few decades ago, relations between mentor and student were deemed indispensable for intergenerational transfer of skills, accumulated wisdom and insights, to learn bedside courtesy and compassion; that learning experience forged lifetime friendships, and collaboration. Today the old-fashioned mentorship has given way to standardized protocols, reliance on technological diagnostics, and the priorities of clinical productivity.

Depersonalized training makes victims of would-be doctors; half of them suffer burnout by the fourth year in medical school. The system fails to prime them to deal with the burden and anguish of caregiving and offers scant comfort and compassion when they stumble. Abraham Verghese, author and physician, has faulted medicine's attitude toward needy physicians as "a silent but terrible collusion to cover up pain, to cover up depression; there is a fear of blushing, a machismo that destroys us." Many doctors avoid ambiguity and are incapable of admitting to the patients that science has blind spots and uncertainties abound in health care. Ludmerer concludes that its own leaders betrayed medicine. As regulators and corporations demanded fiscal discipline, these leaders allied with market interests even as the new ethos subverted medical education and deepened alienation among clinicians and clients.

The same dynamics that have vitiated medical education have leeched human emotion out of caregiving and have rendered the care setting rushed and unsatisfying. To relate and to connect, to love and be loved are quintessentially human traits. Research in long-term care has shown human contact and friendly human exchange are the source of the highest satisfaction and of the greatest motivation for nursing home administrators, the DONs, and all ranks of staff (4.09). The same is true for physicians; 78 percent of them in 2008 said their relationship with the patients was the most satisfying aspect of their practice. Tellingly, that number rose to 80 percent in 2012. It is equally revealing that the second most satisfying aspect of their work was intellectual stimulation for 82 percent in 2008 and for only 70 percent in 2012 (4.10).

Managed care has robbed doctors and nurses of the quintessential reward of their work. As hospitals discharge patients quicker and sicker, physicians get less time to develop relationships with patients and their families. Doctors in training spend only 12.3 percent of their working hours in direct contact with patients. That is, medical residents interact with patients for eight minutes per patient per day. They spend 63.6 percent of their time on indirect patient care, including 20 percent spent on talking to other providers. Computer use took 40 percent, educational activities took 14.7 percent, and 5.9 percent on walking (4.11).

In summary, many obstacles to quality and compassion can be understood at the level of caregiver behavior. It is to be expected that progress and innovation will meet skepticism from many of goodwill. Caregiver behavior often bends to the demands of the system rather than to the dictates of the conscience. When, across health care, commercial ways elbowed out the traditional and humane concerns, leaders in health care failed to protect, preserve, and promote medical training; they stood by and watched the deformation medicine and medical education.

Death's Toll on the Living

The profit motive has been a dominant force in long-term care. OSCAR data shows that of the fifteen thousand nursing homes, 68 percent are run for profit and 55 percent belong to multifacility chains. Consequently, they consider their prime goal is deficiency-free compliance with regulatory norms rather than excellence and person-centered compassionate care.

Nursing homes are notorious for not preparing the new recruits, especially the youngest, to the challenges of their job. This becomes glaringly clear in a salient feature of nursing home life, namely, death and dying. Death is no stranger to a nursing home. Nearly three quarters of a million Americans aged eighty-five or older died in 2007 (i.e., 30 percent of all who died that year in the United States). Among these "very old" who died in 2007, 40 percent died in nursing homes, 29 percent died as hospital inpatients, and 12 percent died while residing at home (4.12). An increasing number of us in an aging America will die in nursing homes. In a span of a month, a CNA is likely to experience four deaths in a typical nursing home.

Unfortunately, training does not teach the CNA to understand and deal with death, mourning, grieving, and associated social rituals. Managers are often oblivious that many of their CNAs come from diverse cultures, classes, and lands and bring to the nursing home their unique approach to death, pain, and suffering. Many nursing homes are less than sensitive to the culture shock CNAs suffer when assigned to help handle the dead body in efficient but sacrilegious ways.

Rarely do nursing homes build on the emotional legacy and friendly bonds that a resident's death leaves behind. Although many nursing homes suffer high CNA turnover, a substantial number hold it below 10 percent. Besides, an average nursing home maintains a solid, stable core: 70 percent of CNAs have served there for more than a year, 15 percent for five to ten years, and 5 percent for over ten years. As for the residents, thirty-five out of one hundred die in the nursing home after an average stay of two years (and are referred to as long-stayers), and thirty-seven spend less than ninety days (the short-stayers) and return to the hospital or home. The data over twelve years clearly show that CNAs and residents develop emotional ties; residents and families highly commend their caregivers (4.13). The ideal type Marge Donovan, profiled in chapter 1, illustrates how the resident-staff bond develops.

Many a manager ignores the hidden potential of these informal ties. Molly, a young CNA, came to work on Monday. Just as it has happened to many other CNAs, Molly was taken aback when she saw a new face in the bed where sweet Martha, her friend, lay when Molly had kissed her good-bye as she went home on Friday. Molly stands there alone with no one who can tell her whether Martha was moved, transferred, or as she suspects, whether she died. She had no opportunity to bid her farewell or to pay her last respects. No one will know her grief. Molly whispers a silent prayer and introduces herself to the ninety-year-old lying in Martha's bed.

Healers in Need of Healing

Every health-care setting, discipline, and rank has its Mollys. The 893,851 practicing physicians are not a happy lot—many are bedeviled by anxiety and worry. One sad statistic provides stark evidence that many members of the healing profession are driven beyond the reach of anyone to heal them. Every year in the United States, over 400 doctors kill themselves—as many doctors as those graduating from two medical schools and a rate twice as high as the general population (4.14).

Physician suicide exceeds the rate for any other profession. It crosses boundaries of medical specialty and income, and it is more lethal (i.e., the completion-to-attempt ratio is higher). Women in medicine suffer a higher rate of major depression than age-matched women with doctorate degrees. Men commit suicide four times more often than women in the general community, but among doctors, the male suicide rate equals the female rate (4.15).

Suicidal doctors lead a troubled life. Two in five doctors who have committed suicide were seeing a mental health professional at the time of death. One in three had at least one psychiatric hospitalization (4. 16). Divorce rate for doctors runs up to 20 percent higher than among the public. They live in more unhappy marriages. About

40 percent of physician suicides are associated with alcoholism and 20 percent with drug abuse (4.16).

Often, a doctor's suicidal journey begins with a baptism of fire in medical school and continues through a harsh socialization. There are 15 to 30 percent of interns who suffer clinical depression, and one in four interns admit having suicidal ideation (4.17).

A relatively recent graduate physician describes her training:

"From my own recent experience in residency [2006], I believe the 'emotional egress' is multifactorial. We most certainly lack empathic and compassionate mentors. While some do exist, they were certainly not the norm in my training institution. Screaming, yelling, demeaning, sarcasm, put-downs, and one-upmanship were the norm for attending and residents, in all of the specialties I saw represented in my large university training program, from medical school through residency. I would not talk to an animal the way these people habitually talk to young, impressionable doctors who are learning from their respected attending.

"The rare kind, thoughtful, professional, courteous attending, who treated students and residents like humans and considered the patient's welfare rather than just their lab values and x-ray reports were demeaned by the sarcastic ones as being incompetent or 'not assertive.'" (4.18).

Suicide is a private event with social origins and consequences. An epidemic of emotional damage, mental anguish, feelings of guilt, depression, and suicide that afflicts caregivers can be explained on the level of personal makeup, choice, and response to the demands of one's vocation and the punishing environment of one's work.

The causal roots of caregiver distress, however, run deeper and stem from the cracks in the foundation of health care. We will address this in the next chapter.

Compassion and Its Discontents

A physician's blog entry in *Ideal Medicine* poignantly summarizes our argument about the triggers of dissatisfaction among doctors (4.19).

> I've been a doctor for twenty years.
> I've not lost a single patient to suicide. I've lost only colleagues, friends, and lovers—ALL male physicians—to suicide.
> Why?
> Here's what I know:
> A physician's greatest joy is the patient relationship.
> Assembly-line medicine undermines the patient-physician relationship.
> Most doctors are burned out, overworked, or exhausted.
> Many doctors spend little time with their families.
> Workaholics are admired in medicine.
> Medicine values competition over nurturing.
> Many doctors function in survival mode.
> Doctors are not supposed to make mistakes.
> Caring for sick people can make you sick if you don't care for yourself.
> Medical education often dissociates mind from body and spirit.
> Some medical students believe they graduate with PTSD.
> Seeing too much pain and not enough joy is unhealthy.
> For a physician, a cry for help is weakness.
> The reductionist medical model is dehumanizing for patient and physician.
> Many doctors are emotionally detached (especially male physicians).

Doctors are obsessive-compulsive perfectionists in an imperfect medical system.

Physicians are the nation's social safety net with few resources to help patients.

Some doctors feel like indentured slaves.

Death is perceived as failure.

Doctors don't take very good care of themselves or each other.

Many doctors are in denial about the high rate of physician suicide.

Physicians are often bullied by insurance companies, employers, and patients.

Doctoring is more than a job; it's a calling, an identity.

Doctors are often socially isolated.

Doctors can't just be people. They're doctors 24/7.

Doctors can feel severe psychological pain.

Doctors can feel powerless.

Doctors can feel trapped. Some see no alternatives to their suffering.

Doctors have easy access to lethal drugs and firearms.

Doctors have the same problems as everyone else.

Doctors have marital distress. They get divorced.

Doctors have addiction to drugs and alcohol.

Doctors have economic hardship and unbearable debt.

Doctors have mental illness.

Doctors are human.

CHAPTER 5
Medicine's Fault Lines

Impediments to Compassion

A harsh paradox lies at the core of modern medicine. Even as it promotes health and cures illness, health care poses a danger to human health. Lucian Leape is the indefatigable crusader for safe, humane medical care (5.01). He extrapolated to all health care in the United States his findings on clinical errors and famously declared that if errors in other industries occurred as often in health care, you would see three jumbo jets crash at Chicago's O'Hare airport every two days, thirty-two thousand checks would be deducted from the wrong bank account every hour, and sixteen thousand pieces of mail would be lost every hour. A profession dedicated to keep us safe and well may in fact harm many.

Part 1. The Enigma of Medicine

This paradox turns into an enigma when you consider that medical errors occur under the watch of its high priests (women and men physicians)—a group that could not be more favored by the gods:

- They are highly educated—minted in demanding academic settings.

- They have ready access to the latest and best medical, pharmaceutical, and human resources.
- They enjoy greater professional autonomy than is the case in most other professions.
- They take pride in their work and walk the extra mile: they do research, they lecture, they publish, and they teach.
- As true professionals, they feel defeated when a treatment does not work; they feel guilty when they make a mistake—even one that does not cause harm.
- They are generous and kind, caring and giving. In 2012, 52 percent of docs gave $35,000 or more uncompensated care (i.e., as charity, patient nonpayment, or denied reimbursement), and 39 percent gave uncompensated care worth $50,000 or more.
- Health care has always appealed to the noble, selfless tendencies in the human heart. Many in health care, from CNAs to physicians, admit feeling called to transcend, to serve, and to give (5.02).

How can a healing profession led by the best, brightest and altruistic practitioners allow patients be victims of their negligence? How can they not know what leads them into such grievous error?

We offered a partial explanation on the level of individual practitioners. The range and seriousness of the errors in caregiving, however, suggest that they could not primarily arise from the stress and strain intrinsic to the vocation of a healer. We will argue that they are the fallout of skewed institutional structures and a flawed culture that prevails in medicine.

The institutional foundation of medicine is potentially at odds with the person-centered values that compassion upholds. Second, health care flouted the advice of the wise Greeks of old. The ancient philosophers preached a truth that history has validated through the centuries: health and well-being are the fruit of a balanced life; to achieve excellence all things have to be in balance. A dynamic system, biological or organizational, carries within it residual flaws of its evolutionary history. In a well-balanced, healthy organism, genetic flaws lie dormant and inactive. Unrestrained behaviors overstrain the system; they turn hairline cracks into gaping fault lines. The upheaval that has shaken modern medicine has brought to light its hidden contradictions and excesses.

To fight a survival war, medicine adopted a harsh strategy that brought it victory and a premier status. That winning strategy included policies and priorities not always aligned with kindness, caring, and compassion. Medicine reengineered itself along rigorous lines. It made clinical education and training stringent and demanding. It severed all ties with holistic health practitioners. It strenuously opposed progressive legislation not conducive to its interests. Furthermore, its unrestrained dominance tempted it to venture off the virtuous middle road of balance and moderation and pushed it to the edge of bigotry, where paradigms turn into dogma, and theory into ideology.

In short, medicine's woes are the legacy of medicine's hard, uncompromising strategies. They constitute the four-layered firewall that impedes the reform. These four obstacles on compassion's pathway can be summarized as the following:

1. Modern medicine disassembles the human person; it fragments the patient, cures the sick body, and leaves the patient, emotionally shaken and stressed in spirit, to fend for oneself.
2. Modern medicine promotes a hierarchy that divides and ranks people; it fosters inequality, inhibits collegiality, and impedes sharing; it diminishes patient autonomy and involvement in self-care.
3. Modern medicine encourages professionalization as a zero-sum game that sorts people into winners and losers;

it reduces trust and changes human relationships into a contractual interchange.

4. Modern medicine has fostered an unreasoned pursuit of specialization that has created specialty enclaves unable to engage in interdisciplinary dialogue, fruitful sharing, and collaboration.

Part 2. Impediments to Compassion

Impediment 1. Medicine Disassembles the Human Person

Science took a giant step forward when the Cartesian dualism gave it a solid theoretical platform. It also boosted evidence-based methodology that resulted in spectacular outcomes in biology.

Dualism challenged the Aristotelian-Aquinas scholastic schema to understand reality; Descartes distinguished physical substance from mental substance, the body from the mind. We can quantify the physical aspects of the body (i.e., size, temperature, weight). The nonphysical attributes of the mind (i.e., thought, beliefs) are beyond our empirical reach. Dualism profoundly altered biology and medicine. Titans like Louis Pasteur and Robert Koch reinforced the dualistic perspective with the germ theory and validated it across the globe by vanquishing humanity's ancient, infectious foes.

The linear causal illness model considers health as the absence of disease, it sees the patient as a passive victim and it expects the practitioner to search for the magic bullet. Such thinking disaggregates the human condition and objectifies human illness and suffering. It depersonalizes the patient and medicalizes life. Over the years, we have witnessed bad breath redefined as halitosis, impotence as erectile dysfunction, and excessive plastic surgery as dysmorphic disorder. The triumph of dualism has been its undoing. A successful scientific methodology has become the central dogma in medicine's orthodoxy—a development that runs contrary to the moderation Descartes refers to in his *Reflections* and practiced by Pasteur and Koch.

Biomedical thinking inhibits the flowering of compassion. It does so, first, by narrowing the mental horizons and putting a mindlock on medical students before they launch their career. Some years ago, I (VT-N) taught a sociology course on alternative modes of healing to medical students at Rush Medical College, Rush University, and Chicago. I brought to the class practitioners of different healing systems—chiropractic, naturopathy, Chinese medicine, reflexology, among others. In each instance, the robust class discussion gave ample evidence of how effectively the medical school had, within two years, molded young minds according to the biomedical model and how confidently those minds screened out contaminating viewpoints.

Young minds shaped by a seductive paradigm retain their doctrinaire bent through years of maturity. My doctor friend, a brain specialist, and I (VT-N) were caught up a in a spirited but friendly dialogue. When I saw an opening, I piloted our conversation toward the effectiveness of alternate modes of healing. Our conversation ended quickly and awkwardly after my friend, the doctor, said with genuine sincerity, untouched by guile, "I am not well acquainted with witches, witchcraft, and witch's brews."

> "Freedom of the mind requires not only the absence of legal constraints but the presence of alternative thoughts. The most successful tyranny is not the one that uses force to assure uniformity, but the one that removes awareness of other possibilities."
> —*Alan Bloom,* The Closing of the American Mind *(1987)*

Much of medical school reform is seed sown on rocky fields. "We cannot solve our problems with the same kind of thinking that created them," Albert Einstein had observed commonsensically. He could have well been referring to schools that train our health-care practitioners. The biomedical paradigm guides and gives direction to the curriculum and pedagogy in every type of clinical training. It cuts the heart out of incompatible innovations and leaves behind an empty shell.

The case of continuing education of physicians serves as an example. New requirements for the Maintenance of Certification (MOC) of medical specialties prescribes that every physician be recertified every ten years by passing a costly exam; those who do not risk being tagged as uncertified. Recertification has become its own industry, and its "practice assessments" just onerous paperwork, says Danielle Ofri, MD. The biomedical bias favors scientific knowledge—narrowly defined. She commented, "There is much more to the science, art, and practice of medicine than medical knowledge... Memorizing reams of information to be regurgitated in a 'secure testing center' is a waste of time and resources." It may even divert one from the cultivation and practice of compassion.

Biomedicine undercuts compassion in a second way. In the case of Harold Maxwell, the ideal type profiled in chapter 2, biomedicine depersonalized him; it split him in two and expertly set about to repair his body. It gave no thought to Harold the person. It ignored how his illness had damaged his psyche, had made him afraid, insecure, tense, and anxious; it was unconcerned that his near-death experience had strained his family relations. The caregiver team stood by, knowing full well that his emotional turmoil and his family's distress would set back Harold's recovery.

Interviews and history-taking are the basis for diagnostics and treatment. The care team, however, had no clue about Harold's personal and clinical biography. The fact that the art of history-taking is fast becoming a lost art (5.03), it diminishes the humanity of the surgeon and her support team. They had to stand by and let Harold wrestle with his demons. The surgeon had to remind herself that she was primarily a clinical engineer; her profession judged her by her clinical success and not by the compassion she brought to the operating table. In fact, she better not step out of her specialized role and risk liability by extending a helping hand without appropriate credentials.

Health care failed Harold in yet another way—it unnecessarily limited his choices. Harold had expected a university-based hospital would offer him complementary therapeutics. In 2007, 38 percent of adults used CAM. Eighty-three million American adults spent $33.9 billion out of pocket on CAM, i.e., 11.2 percent of total out-of-pocket expenditures on health care (5.04). About 42 percent of hospitals offer at least one CAM therapy (5.05). Unfortunately, Harold Maxwell did not benefit by the positive change occurring in hospitals.

In another instance, he put his unwell heart at risk and let himself get angry when the hospital deprived him of a visit from his father confessor and spiritual guide. Harold is a Catholic; religion and spirituality are a big part of his life. The hospital not only showed unconcern for Harold's spiritual needs but its biomedicalized culture also seemed oblivious to common wisdom that the human mind and the human spirit are effective healers as well as killers. They can heal much more surely than the most potent potion in the pharmacopeia. The worry beads of Islamic cultures, the rosary beads of the Catholic Church, the spiritual exercises of the Jesuit Founder St. Ignatius—all these practices may have greater curative power than does the relaxation response, whose potential has been established by Harvard researchers. All this is alien land to clinicians who are averse to mix the spiritual with the clinical; rarely do clinicians have the skill and tools to draw on religion for healing.

The biomedical bias marginalizes religious experience of patients. A total of 78 percent of Americans admit being religious. Catholics are the largest denominational group in the United States, constituting 20.8 percent of the population. Mainline denominational Protestants total 14.7 percent, denominational evangelicals add up to 25.4 percent, and black church members make up 6.5 percent (5.06).

Religion rises in importance in times of crises, uncertainty, and illness:

- There are 65 percent of patients who wish doctors talked with them about their spiritual beliefs.
- Two out of three place greater trust in a doctor who is tuned into their spiritual concerns.
- There are 94 percent of patients whose spiritual beliefs are important to them and who want their physicians to be sensitive to their spiritual needs.
- There are 95 percent of cancer patients who draw on their spiritual beliefs, and 49 percent became more spiritual after their diagnosis.

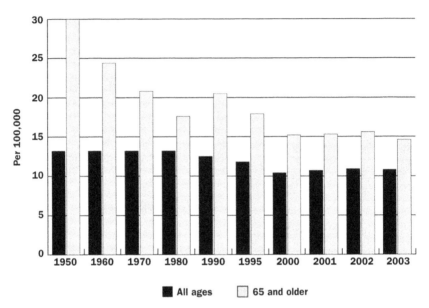

Suicides All vs. Elderly 1950–2003: USA

Yet only 10 percent say a doctor has talked with them about their spiritual faith as a factor related to their physical health. (5.07).

Harold Koenig, director of Duke University's Center for Spirituality, Theology, and Health, has been engaged since 2010 in a study involving several hundred patients treated with therapeutic approaches rooted in Christianity, Islam, Judaism, Hinduism, and Buddhism (5.08). In his 2004 review of research on the impact of religion on humans, especially when they are ill, he concluded that the spiritually conflicted are significantly more likely to die during the posthospital follow-up period. For every one-point increase on a religious struggles scale, mortality increases 6 percent—independent of physical health, social support, and psychological status. Religious people tend to be healthier mentally and physically. Religion adds about seven years to the life span of white people and about fourteen years to the lives of people in ethnic minorities. In the university-af-filiated hospital, Harold's right to autonomy, choice, and preference in matters of religion and healing ritual did not register on the radar screen.

The nursing home, however, was surprisingly well tuned to Harold's religious desires. An interdisciplinary team designed his care plans, which included his religious preferences. He attended Sunday mass, celebrated by a kindly priest assisted by an ancient-looking nun in her traditional antique habit. Harold was the lector. He exuded comfort and joy reading aloud the First Epistle of Paul the apostle to the Corinthians, chapter 1 and verses 1 to 13. "Though I speak with the tongues of men and of angels, and have not charity, I am become as sounding brass, or a tinkling cymbal."

Thus, the biomedical dualism that brought many blessings to humanity tuned into an ideology out of step with compassion. It trained practitioners that could not handle matters of mind and spirit.

Impediment 2. Medical Inequality Degrades the Person

Inequality and stratification are endemic to medicine. You can see them in every area of health care in the open or under a thousand guises. In every manifestation, inequality stands at the opposite extreme of compassion. Inequality breeds hierarchies of status, privilege, and power; it sorts individuals into superiors and subordinates; and it tends to monopolize, dominate, and exploit.

Compassion and mutual caring, on the other hand, thrive where people are equal, empathize, and relate. Compassion tunes in to the wavelength of the other, enters the other's personal world, and shares the trouble and pain of the other. If joy shared equals joy doubled, a pain shared is pain halved. Compassion is the greatest healer. Equality is its greatest catalyst.

We will track the ways of inequality, how we unwittingly endorse it, and the ugly trail it leaves behind in health care. And harms us all.

Wordless Clues Broadcast Your Rank

Inequality of class, rank, and rewards is a fact of life, but it is particularly incongruent in a compassionate, healing environment. In ways both blatant and unobtrusive, hierarchy, status, and privilege manifest themselves at every level, from the doctor-patient encounters to the institutional operations.

We (VT-N and MT-N) conducted an ethnographic study of how unequals interact in the hospital. Our intent was to document how everyday manners, courtesies, and etiquette reflect the social inequalities that are the stuff of life. (5.09).

We observed life on the hospital floor at different sites, where rank separates doctors and nurses into different status groups. Their job requires the two groups to collaborate and communicate; at the same time, inequality demands that the two parties maintain a social distance as befits their unequal status. Doctors and nurses rely on body language and social rituals that not only let them cooperate as a team but also to silently announce to the world they are truly unequals.

Thus, a woman nurse steps up and unobtrusively rescues a medical resident from a tight spot, but her demeanor, voice, and choice of words make it obvious that she defers to the doctor's authority. Both physician and nurse use behavioral codes and symbols that leave no doubt who holds the higher rank.

Humans love inequality, so we have created hundreds of props to display our social rank to others. At every turn, wordless clues broadcast your rank to the world: the size and location of your office, the time you spend waiting in line; the tone of your voice, the delay of your response when questioned, the firmness of your handshake, the extent of the personal space that separates you when talking to subordinates, how attentively you listen, when and whom you interrupt, with whom you make direct eye contact, and in whose presence you feel free to slouch.

Recall Diane Schneider, our second ideal type, and watch inequality in action in the doctor-patient visit. Inequality sets the direction for the interaction and guides it along an unwritten but established protocol. At the start, the doctor holds the monopoly over assets of high value—knowledge and skills. Class and status add another dimension to the doctor-patient disparity. Illness sharpens its edge and renders the patient dependent, vulnerable, anxious, and sometimes, thoroughly shaken. The advantage tilts totally in favor of the physician.

Physicians often are unaware that a social gulf separates them from the patient; many patients view doctors as omnipotent, look at them with awe; feeling dependent and insecure, they search for a meaning in the doctor's slightest smile, in the tone of the voice, or in an inadvertent gesture.

The gentlemanly Dr. Murphy, although known for his old-fashioned politeness and courtesies, still failed to read the subtext in the story of his shaken patient. She saw unconcern and aloofness in his body language. The encounter was a waste of time, money, and opportunity. It set back Diane's purpose, and Dr. Murphy, oblivious of the turmoil he had unwittingly created, moved on to the next appointment and, perhaps, to another clinical fiasco.

How often have you seen a doctor or nurse sitting by the bedside engaged in a conversation with a patient? How often have you seen a patient explaining what ails her or him, while the nurse or doctor interrupts, keeps tapping the pencil, places a hand on the door handle, avoids eye contact, or scrolls up and down on the computer screen? These gestures silently assert hierarchy: who is in charge, whose time has greater value, and who can violate rules of courtesy.

The patient reads the nonverbal message: the nurse or doctor is not concerned, has no time for personal details, and above all, do not expect empathy or sympathy. In surveys, six in ten doctors say medical school had poorly prepared them to talk to patients (5.10).

Most doctors fail to see and appreciate how a face-to-face office visit can intimidate a vulnerable patient. Consider this suggestion: the training of doctors and nurses should include power-swapping exercises. How would an office visit feel like, if in a wardrobe swap, the patient was attired as a Wall Street executive and the doctor wore the patient's paper gown—an apt symbol of vulnerability, dependence, and powerlessness.

Thus, our daily informal social interaction is not as spontaneous and free as we may think. Just as we follow rules of grammar in formal speech, so too we unknowingly follow the strict grammar of body language that conforms to the rules of inequality. Every moment our posture, attire, demeanor and gestures display and reinforce hierarchy and stratification nowhere as surely and with negative outcomes as in health care.

Inequality Sets Stage for Abuse

Pauline W. Chen, MD, writes about the rude streaks in the medical culture doctor's experience early in medical school (5.10).

"Powerfully built and with the face of a boxer, he cast a bone-chilling shadow wherever he went in the hospital… The young man was a brilliant and promising young doctor who took his patients' conditions to heart but who also possessed a temper so explosive that medical students dreaded working with him. He had called various classmates 'stupid' and 'useless' and could erupt with little warning in the middle of hospital halls. Like frightened little mice, we endured the treatment as an inevitable part of medical training, fearful that doing otherwise could result in a career-destroying evaluation or grade.

"But one day, one of our classmates, having already been on the receiving end of several of this doctor's tirades, shouted back. She questioned one of his conclusions in front of the rest of the medical team, insisted on getting an explanation, and then screamed back when he started yelling at her.

"The entire episode unnerved us all; and over the next few weeks, we marveled at her courage and fretted over her potentially ruined career prospects. But there was one aspect of the event that disturbed us even more. One classmate who had witnessed the 'screaming match' described how our fellow medical student had raised her voice and positioned her body as she threatened the doctor. 'It was weird,' he recounted. 'It was like watching her turn into him.'

"Becoming a doctor requires more than an endless array of standardized exams, long hours on the wards, and years spent in training. For many medical students, verbal and physical harassment and intimidation are part of the exhausting process, too."

Social imbalance sets the stage for inequality; power imbalance provides the temptation to turn inequality into abuse. Much of medical training occurs in a setting that is both an occasion and a temptation for abusive behavior.

K. Silver, MD, worked with abused children and revealed to the world, in 1990, the ugly face of inequity and inhumanity built into the curriculum of a medical student (5.11). *JAMA* published his revelation that, on average, 46 percent of students are abused in medical school, and by their senior year, 81 percent of them suffer abuse. About 69 percent of these victims described that experience as of "major importance and very upsetting." Its adverse effect lasted for a month or more for 49.6 percent, while 16 percent expected it would "always affect them." Medical students said they were yelled at, pushed, and threatened. One student was slapped on the hand by a senior doctor, who said, "If teaching doesn't help you learn, then pain will." Another student said, "A surgical resident threatened to kill me during a chest tube placement." Some endured insults, mocking by senior staff making noises to mimic a foreign language, being grabbed, being asked out on a date, or being passed over because of their gender.

Disrespectful behavior in health care takes many forms: angry outbursts, verbal threats, shouting, swearing; threat or actual infliction of unwarranted physical force; temper tantrum, throwing objects, breaking things; unwanted physical contact of a sexual nature; profane, disrespectful, insulting or abusive language; loud or inappropriate arguments, demeaning comments or intimidation; shaming others for negative outcomes; simple rudeness and gratuitous negative comments; severe judgment or censuring colleagues or staff in front of patients, visitors, or other staff; bullying; insensitive comments about a patient's medical condition, appearance, or situation; and jokes or nonclinical comments about race, ethnicity, religion, sexual orientation, age, physical appearance, or socioeconomic or educational status. Such treatment also occurs in the preclinical classroom or laboratory, but it is more common in clinical settings like hospital wards or clinics.

Bullying Culture

Abuse in the training years does not occur at random. It is rooted in and encouraged by the cultural values accepting of unkindness. Medical schools divide people into groups with unequal status and authority and provide higher-ups unique advantage and give them tenured employment. Academic freedom shields them; they feel invincible as high-revenue producers and feel secure behind the professional and political firewalls they have erected over the years. An impregnable bunker instills fear of retaliation, discourages reporting, and makes improbable the confronting and disciplining of bullying behavior.

Power warps one's viewpoint and portrays dependents as underlings, be they students, junior doctors, interns, nurses, CNAs, and other vulnerable groups. Vulnerability of the subordinate and the invulnerability of the superior make the former easy targets of disrespect, mistreatment, harassment, humiliation, unreasonable demands, and pressure. A hierarchical culture looks benignly on mis-use of power.

Disrespectful behavior becomes a survival strategy for some— they learn to be aggressive enough to discourage anyone from going after them. This initiates a *cycle of abuse*. Mistreated students become doctors who mistreat other medical students. Over the years, this cycle of abuse becomes a part of the culture and the hidden curriculum (5.12).

In Silver's study, medical residents were the worst offenders: they caused 40 percent of the total abuse, 36 percent of sexual harassment, and 26 percent of the physical harm. Clinical faculty was a close second: they caused 36 percent of the total damage, 36 percent of the sexual harassment, and 36 percent of physical abuse.

In 1995, the David Geffen School of Medicine at the University of California, Los Angeles, began to institute school-wide reforms to prevent medical student mistreatment. It instituted safe mechanisms for reporting mistreatment, it provided resources for discussion and resolution, and it educated faculty and residents on the subject. The school logged the incidence, severity, and sources of perceived mistreatment over the thirteen-year period during which the reform measures were implemented. In 2012, the medical school published the results of the effort. They are a severe indictment of modern medicine (5.13).

The bullying culture had hardly changed. A sizable number of medical students still said that they had been mistreated. About 36 percent of male students suffered verbal abuse (a decline of 22 percentage points), and 42 percent of females suffered verbal abuse (a decline of 10 percentage points). Power abuse declined about 16 percent for both males and females. The rate of physical abuse for men was half the rate for women and fell slightly, while it doubled for women. About 10 percent were physically hurt. Sexual harassment more than doubled for men and decreased by 11 percent points for women. "We were really crushed when we saw the results," said Joyce M. Fried, lead author of the paper and assistant dean and chairwoman of the Gender and Power Abuse Committee at the medical school. "We were disappointed that it was so difficult to change."

The Wages of Disrespect

A culture that accommodates inequality and tolerates disrespect does much worse than hurt the victim. It increases the risk of clinical error and harms the patient. In 2008, 4,500 nurses, physicians, and other health-care professionals from 102 hospitals responded to a survey. About 70 percent said disrespect leads to errors, 65 percent said it leads to adverse events, and more than 25 percent linked intimidation to patient mortality (5.14)!

The Institute for Safe Medication Practices (ISMP) studied workplace intimidation and surveyed nurses, pharmacists, physicians, and other health professionals. Of those who were concerned about a medication order, 40 percent had avoided meeting with the intimidating prescriber by dispensing the medication or asking another professional to alert the prescriber. Almost half were pressured to dispense a medication despite their concerns about the order. In the prior year, 7 percent had taken part in a medication error involving intimidation. It was not uncommon to hear a doctor respond sternly, "Just give what I ordered." Some were explicitly threatening, some used condescending language or tone, and some showed impatience when questioned (19 percent). Almost half of the respondents (49 percent) suffered strong verbal abuse at least once during the last year. Pharmacists experienced intimidation more frequently than nurses (5.15).

In 2009, the American College of Physician Executives surveyed 2,100 physicians and nurses (5.16). The physicians and nurses admitted a fundamental lack of respect between the two groups. Nearly 85 percent indicated that disrespect took form of degrading comments and insults, followed by yelling (73 percent), cursing (49 percent), and inappropriate joking (46 percent).

"The worst behavior problem is not the most egregious," added one respondent. "It's the everyday lack of respect and communication that most adversely affects patient care and staff morale" (5.17). One nurse recalled a case in which a nurse had called a patient's physician several times to ask him to go into the intensive care unit (ICU) to see a patient whose condition was declining. Each time, the physician became verbally abusive and refused to go into the hospital. After two attempts, the nurse hesitated to call the physician again despite the patient's continued deterioration. By the time she called again, the patient was hemorrhaging internally, was rushed to the operating room, and then died. Disrespect makes the workplace unfriendly and hinders communication, adversely affecting patient care.

Theresa Brown, RN, refers to a nurse's vulnerable position and the mistreatment she suffered (5.18).

"The most damaging bullying is not flagrant and does not fit the stereotype of a surgeon having a tantrum in the operating room. It is passive, like not answering pages or phone calls, and tends toward the subtle: condescension rather than outright abuse, and aggressive or sarcastic remarks rather than straightforward insults... The bad behavior of even a few of them can set a corrosive tone for the whole organization. Nurses in turn bully other nurses, attending physicians bully doctors-in-training, and experienced nurses sometimes bully the newest doctors."

A Susan J. Behrens, Brooklyn, May 8, 2011, posted the following blog in *The New York Times* on disrespectful behavior in hospitals (5.19):

> Of course nurses aren't the only target of doctor-bullying. Patients, too, cannot guarantee that their doctors will treat them as equals. And sometimes they can be patronized in front of strangers.
>
> During my stint as a linguistic researcher at a rather famous Northeastern hospital, I attended daily rounds for new doctors. One (memorable) morning, the attending physician was proudly displaying to his audience all the skills that had been lost by an elderly man who had recently suffered a stroke. "Look at how he cannot repeat after me, how he has trouble holding up two fingers, now three fingers," and so on.
>
> The doctor then filled a small cup with water and asked the patient to slowly raise it and drink from it, all the time winking at us that he wouldn't be able to do so. The cup got halfway to the patient's mouth, at which point revenge was had: he tossed the water all over the physician.

An authoritative panel of seven experienced experts, including Lucian L. Leape, MD, six other notable physicians, and one health-care executive, summed up the role of disrespect in medicine: "Disrespectful behavior is the root cause of the dysfunctional culture that permeates health care and stymies progress in safety. It is also a product of that culture" (5.20).

Impediment 3. Medicine Promotes Disengaged Professionalism

Professionalization is the hallmark of modernity and a fault line in modern medicine.

In everyday parlance, professionalism conveys two meanings. In the context of specialization, professionalization refers to a select group that has knowledge and mastery over a particular aspect of health care. In a second sense, professionalization refers to the cardinal virtue of a scientist—namely, objectivity. A practitioner's self-image includes the ability to be objective and disciplined, to set aside personal feelings and bias, and to eschew emotional ties and relationships.

Medicine's Pledge to Society

In the classic view, a profession is an occupational group that has won public trust and gained state approval to operate in an exclusive area. Society confers on a profession the right to admit recruits, to set standards, to enforce compliance to them by its members, and to self-police member behavior (5.21).

Society and the state confer these rights and privileges on the group because its members are self-disciplined, highly trained, and have exclusive expertise in an area beneficial to the community. On its part, the group professes (publicly declares) that it will provide those services to the community.

This social contract between medicine and the public is not always in writing, not always crystallized in its obligations and scope. The mutual pledge is a roughly balanced reciprocal exchange. The two sides readjust the agreement when circumstances change. If medics fall short of what the public expects, society may lower reimbursement or make stringent regulation. On the other hand, when red tape and paperwork become burdensome, health care may refuse to serve Medicare or Medicaid patients.

There is no central regulatory body for doctors. State medical boards license doctors, investigate complaints, and discipline those who break the law. An umbrella organization called the American Board of Medical Specialties (ABMS) maintains the standards for the certification of the most common specialties and subspecialties.

The ABMS was formed in 1933, when health care boasted four approved specialties. They numbered ten in 1935 and increased to twenty in the 1970s. In 2013, ABMS listed 159 specialties and 29 subspecialties. Several specialty societies are waiting in the wings to be approved, and many more are sprouting in the health-care field (5.22). Approved specialties in nursing 76 and poised to grow in numbers (5.23).

Many professions nest subspecialties within them. Typically, each is associated with an ever-narrowing specialty, and each seeks a distinctive identity, with its own name, colors, logo, and image. Each sets up its own formal association, offers its own accreditation, publishes its own journals, develops its own jargon, holds its own conventions, and charges dues.

In effect, a new profession adds yet a new silo to a landscape crowded with such silos. In keeping with its evolutionary history, medicine as a profession has assumed a competitive posture and has made ramparts of these silos. Medicine has played a zero-sum game:

for one to win, the other has to lose. A group rises in professional status at the expense of another group. Turf battles often end up in court. Rivalry curbs professional interchange, sharing, and dialogue.

By the first half of the twentieth century, allopathic medicine had emerged as a clear victor vis-à-vis rival healers and healing systems. Most were wiped off the map. A few survived in the deep shadows. Of these, osteopathy got in the good graces of medicines, and chiropractic became the main target of witch hunts. Back in 1911, the AMA's hostility was epitomized in *Nostrums and Quackery*, which ranted against quackery and medical fraud as "forces of evil," led by "misguided fakers" (5.24). That exclusionist fervor continued through the decades and demanded that a physician should not voluntarily associate professionally with anyone with a practice without a scientific basis. In 1964, the AMA instituted the Committee on Quackery. In 1996, Stephen Barrett founded Quackwatch, a network that combats health-related frauds, myths, fads, fallacies, and unproven or ineffective healing methods.

Medicine's self-identity as the only legitimate and science-based clinical profession meshes well with the exclusionist biomedical model. Together they construct cul-de-sacs that isolate these professionals from professionals of other persuasion. Absence of bridges across professions stymies efforts to build integrative medicine, cross-fertilization of knowledge, and maximization of consumer choice.

This isolationist, chauvinistic approach is antipathetic to the outsider blocks cooperation, collaboration sharing that compassion preaches. This overt negative attitude filters down to many other health-related professions. The training of nurses, pharmacists, rehab therapists, and of others, imparts a bio-medical mind-set skeptical of compassion.

On the level of interaction with clients, the equinamitas expected of a clinical professional dampens rather than encourages empathy and compassion. Empathy ushers you into the private world of another and lets you view life from that person's eyes. Compassion takes the next step and makes you feel the pain the other experiences.

Medicine has made compassion a hard virtue to practice. A clinician is pulled in two directions. On one side, your profession places high value on and rewards self-assurance, stoicism, and emotional disengagement; on the other side, compassion calls you to reach out, to feel for and to suffer with the patient. Many nurses and physicians have buckled under such a tension. Research has shown that those who display great compassion are at greater risk for compassion fatigue (5.25). One nurse wrote, "I have felt compassion fatigue when caring for a young, dying cancer patient. No words I offer or medications I give would change the outcome. Daily I watched this patient's youthful personality decline."

The victims of compassion fatigue lose the balance between altruism and self-care; they forget the boundary between duty and sacrifice; they internalize patient's woes beyond their ability to handle the burden. Their training did not teach them to savor the rewards of compassion or to detect the dangers of stifling compassion or to balance the dictates of the professional code and the call of compassion.

Caring Touch with a Gloved Hand

Medicine has elevated the image of the professional in the public mind. A professional stands out from the others by her or his expert knowledge or skill, by the high standards of personal ethics, and is expected to deliver a quality product.

At the same time, the professionalism that medicine has advocated and rewarded embraces and practices biomedical principles. Its ideal is the professional who is an expert in matters of the body, unemotional, detached, and prefers a high-tech cure over healing with a caring touch, personal connection, and compassion.

Medicine's detached, impersonal competitive professionalism has discouraged dialogue and sharing between disciplines; it has replaced the caring touch with the sterile contact of the gloved hand.

Detachment starves personal relationships, which are so paramount in life, more so in health care and most so in a nursing home. As happened in the case of Marge Donavon, our ideal type in chapter 2, friendly exchange calms the agitated new resident, makes the lonely or anxious elderly feel secure. The most effective language of social relationship is the universal, primal mother tongue, the healing language of touch.

History, research, and anecdote have amply shown that the caring touch has magical therapeutic effects. It eases pain, helps infant growth, stabilizes body temperature, strengthens relationships, fortifies the immune system, releases serotonin, stimulates oxytocin (the cuddle hormone), slows heart rate, lowers blood pressure, lowers the stress hormone cortisol, gives comfort, relieves sadness, brings joy, reduces migraine pain, and induces sleep.

It is both realistic and profoundly symbolic that nurses in hospitals wear gloves routinely; nurses in nursing homes use them for specific clinical procedures.

The best-selling author and professor of medicine at Stanford University Abraham Verghese describes with a lyricist's touch the spiritual chemistry that is created when the doctor's hands examine the body of the patient (5.26):

> When we are sick, we become infantilized; we seek the reassuring touch of the surrogate father or mother, the only ones who can touch us with impunity and bring about laughter and comfort. A careful [physical] exam invokes the

mythic rites of priest and confessant, of saint and disciple, of healer and sufferer. In these modern times, when medical care is so fractured, a thorough exam conveys attentiveness in addition to providing comfort and reassurance. At the end of this ritual, physician and patient are no longer strangers but are bonded through touch, and yet the ritual is fully connected with the science and knowledge of our time. That bond moves the patient toward healing—not just of the body, but of the psychic wound, that accompanies physical illness. I don't want to imply that the bedside exam is only about ritual; for me and other physicians of a certain age and training, it remains an invaluable diagnostic tool, one that puts us a day or two ahead of those who have to rely on imaging and other tests before they can make a move. But it's nice to realize what else the exam does.

Research shows that physical affection has measurable health benefits. Stimulating touch receptors under the skin can lower blood pressure and cortical levels, effectively reducing stress. One study from the University of North Carolina found that women who hugged their spouse or partner frequently (even for just twenty seconds) had lower blood pressure, possibly because a warm embrace increases oxytocin levels in the brain. As a noted neurologist puts it, "A hug, pat on the back and even a friendly handshake are processed by the reward center in the central nervous system, which is why they can have a powerful impact on the human psyche, making us feel happiness and joy. And it doesn't matter if you're the toucher or touchee. The more you connect with others—on even the smallest physical level—the happier you'll be."

Research at UC Berkeley's School of Public Health found that a doctor making eye contact and giving a pat on the back from a doctor may boost survival rates of patients with complex diseases. Research has also shown that sympathetic touch from a doctor during visit makes such a positive impression that the patient remembers the visit to have lasted twice as long as untouched patients say about their visit (5.27).

In sum, competitive, dispassionate professionalism has made the physician–patient bond sterile, making it difficult for it to coexist with compassion.

Impediment 4. Specialists Isolated in Silos

We think of an ideal physician as one who is broadly informed on medical matters, who understands your illness in the big picture, who knows you and your family, who listens and who engages you in your care. That describes a primary care physician, the kind we all desire to have but have ever-greater difficulty in finding because medicine seems intent on turning out not caring doctors and nurses but narrowly specialized, dispassionate, and unengaged bioengineers.

Erosion of Primary Care

Medicine's pursuit of technologically adept specialists has come at the price of the erosion of primary care and of the retreat of compassion into the shadows.

"Unfortunately, less than 15 percent of graduating medical students will be in primary care practices," reported University of Georgia professor Mark Ebell in 2009 (5.28). "In most countries, about half of students are in primary care practices, and those countries consistently have better health outcomes and provide care more efficiently than in the U.S." Many countries have developed strong primary care infrastructures. Britain has integrated primary and hospital-based care. Canada has only 10 percent more specialists than primary care physicians, in contrast to over 50 percent more in the USA (5.29).

One physician bemoaned, "We in primary care are suffering from a death of a thousand cuts of indignities. I would NEVER recommend any physician go into primary care today" (5.30).

Experts estimate that 75 percent to 85 percent of Americans need only primary care services in a given year; 10 percent to 12 percent require referrals to short-term secondary care services; 5 percent to 10 percent use tertiary care services. Medicine, however, is racing in the opposite direction. In the decade of 2001 and 2010, medical students in the United States increased by 13.6 percent, but those entering primary care fields decreased by 6.3 percent (5.31).

As medicine splinters into ever narrower specialties, cracks appear in the cornerstone of health care: the doctor-patient bond forged in face-to-face encounters—about 150,000 during a physician's career. A therapeutic bond arises when a clinician gets to know the person inside the patient. A good physician considers a patient as a unique person with a unique history and explores it through an open-ended inquiry, shows respect, listens without interruption, relies on human touch to diagnose and to reassure. A good physician will not delegate a nurse or a PA to conduct such an old-fashioned healing ritual. This did not happen in the case of the Diane-Murphy office visit illustrated in our second ideal type in chapter 2.

Malpractice is both a symptom and a result of the breakdown of communication between doctor and patient. As early in 1973, 71 percent of the malpractice claims were shown to result from poor physician-patient relationship. Most litigious patients perceived their physicians as uncaring. One in four found them to be poor communicators, while 13 percent described them as poor listeners (5.32).

Good doctor-patient communication affects how patients adhere to the prescribed regimen and learn self-management. One in three patients do not inform their doctor that they underuse medication for chronic conditions. At discharge from hospital, less than half of patients know their diagnosis or their medications. (5.33)

The length and quality of doctor-patient communication drive malpractice liability. Office visits reduce liability when the physician listens actively to the patient, does not control the agenda, pays attention to the patient's emotional needs, shows empathy in verbal and body language, solicits the patient's viewpoint, and gets agreement on goal of visit and medical care.

Communication and the Most Egregious Error

A supreme irony lies in the fact that as the world takes giant strides in communication and social networking, a communication breakdown stalks health care. Communication is the lifeline of modern life. Miscommunication is the bane of health care. It kills, maims, and inflicts pain. Rapid specialization has led to unfortunate disjunctures within health care.

A wit summarized what you can expect when unedifying rush to professionalize occurs on the heels of unreasoned specialization: "A specialist is one who knows more and more about less and less, till he knows everything about nothing."

In response to the IOM 1999 revelation that hospitals make unconscionable number of avoidable mistakes, President Clinton's task force set about identifying the root of medical error and its prevention (5.34). It quickly reached a conclusion that was endorsed by most experts. The task force repeatedly stressed the central role of communication, collaboration, and teamwork in ensuring patient safety.

Specialization exacts a horrific price when a hospital invests in state-of-the-art safety paraphernalia but fails to cultivate interpersonal bonds, sharing, and communication. Research in the first decade of this century shows that ineffective team communication caused nearly 66 percent of all medical errors for that period (5.35).

The most egregious error in medicine resulting from a failure of communication occurs when a surgical team of credentialed experts wields the scalpel on the wrong person, the wrong organ, the wrong limb, or the wrong vertebra. Patients go to the hospital looking for cures but end up as victims of miscommunication.

Wrong-site surgery (WSS) occurs in the USA about forty times a week according to The Joint Commission. Another study reported that WSSs constitute 1.8 percent of orthopedic surgical claims. WSS most commonly occurs in orthopedic or podiatric procedures, general surgery, and urological and neurosurgical procedures (5.36).

Reported wrong-site surgery (WSS) has increased in recent years; the reported WSS may be only 10 percent of the actual occurrence, cautions The Joint Commission. From the inception of The Joint Commission's Sentinel Event program, the number of WSSs reported has increased from 15 cases in 1998 to 592 cases reported by June 30, 2007. About 79 percent of wrong-site eye surgery and 84 percent of wrong-site orthopedic claims resulted in malpractice awards (5.37).

In 2003, The Joint Commission convened a summit, including leaders from twenty-three other organizations, to address the continued escalation of reported WSS. A major outcome of the summit was creation of a protocol, the Universal Protocol for Preventing Wrong Site. Some recommendations by The Joint Commission:

- Mark the operative site and involve the patient in this process.
- Require oral verification of the correct site in the operating room by each member of the surgical team.
- Follow a verification checklist that includes all documents and medical records referencing the intended operative procedure and site. Directly involve the operating surgeon in the informed consent process.

Silos that specialists inhabit, however, are akin to marbles in a pouch; they touch but do not relate or communicate or share. How well will the Universal Protocol forestall risk? We will address this question in the chapters below.

To conclude, medicine's history and legacy have led to unintended after-effects that have exiled kindness and humanity. The following chapters offer a humanistic framework to better understand the invisible firewalls against compassion and a humanistic pathway for its return.

Part 3. Exemplars of Resident Empowerment

You've heard enough lectures and homilies on empowerment of staff and residents. Now you should go to Bethel, Connecticut, and visit Bethel Health and Rehabilitation Center and the Cascades Assisted Living. In this nursing home, nestled in a twenty-five-acre wooded site, a quietly smart DON, Diane Judson, has incarnated the concept of empowerment in a remarkably simple form that yields unusually big results.

Judson does not hire her CNAs anymore—the residents do. You would expect the DON to be involved in every aspect of recruiting a CNA, and Judson is indeed involved. But at the hour of decision, she silently steps aside, and the residents take over.

Dialogue across Generations

A team of four to six residents, their homework done and ready to meet the applicant, strolled into the conference room. It was a meeting of the ages. On one side was arrayed the accumulated wisdom of the seniors, who looked benignly across the table at the eager young aspirant, Angelica Riviera, nineteen, idealistic but nervous. The dialogue across generations continued for forty-five minutes with storytelling, jokes, and much laughter, as each side wondered how the other side would affect its future.

Proceedings such as these do not always go smoothly. At one point in this example, Robert Murray, a resident on the recruiting panel, pushed Angelica to the emotional edge; she was in tears. Murray asked her, "Angelica, you see, I am only forty-two, but I am not a whole person anymore. Lou Gehrig's ALS has crippled me. I can barely move around. I cannot talk with you without this amplifier headset. I was a full person once. I am not anymore. Angelica, as my caregiver, what can you do to make me feel whole again?"

"That is not what I had expected," Angelica told us. "I thought they would ask me about my training, my skills, and my experience. Bob's question cut through all that I anticipated, it went deep inside me. It told me that what they were looking for was not a CNA. They wanted a caregiver that made them feel like a whole person. I cried."

The recruiting team got the insight they were seeking. Angelica is now a caregiver at Bethel—a happy one. The team has shown an uncanny and unerring insight—how much sensitivity and kindness an applicant brings to the job. Not all applicants pass the test. Of the forty or so prospective students or CNAs thus screened by the residents and recruited in the past year, only two have left Bethel; one was hired by Judson against the team's recommendation—she soon discovered they were right—and the other, although big in heart, fell short on competence.

Above All, Compassion

Murray, the resident afflicted with ALS for six years, has been very active in recruiting CNAs. I asked him what prime qualities he and his mates look for in a prospective CNA. Without hesitation and with emotion, he replied, "Compassion, empathy, and competence"—a succinct summary of what researchers have heard residents repeatedly tell them.

We should not miss the irony. In long-term care, we ardently advocate staff adequacy and competence; we keep inventing ways to measure them. However, we do not measure compassion and empathy, the two things that research shows are the marks of quality and what residents truly desire.

Judson, a thirty-year veteran in health care, has left her mark in many settings. As a successful leader, she is tuned in to her residents and her staff. Once, Barbara Habekost, a seventy-six-year-old resident, casually mentioned to Judson how much she wished that her caregiver (a CNA who was doing her internship at Bethel) would continue to be her caregiver. Inside Judson, a seed sprouted and blossomed into a program allowing residents to choose their own caregivers.

"Seeing residents hire their caregivers is rewarding enough," says Judson. "It has also elevated my understanding of what matters most to the residents. It has made me a better leader and a better person. It is an empowering and uniting experience for us all. Sitting on the sidelines, I listen to residents tell a budding caregiver what living in a facility is all about. At each session, I learn something new."

The Learning Curve

The residents on the Bethel recruiting team are also riding the learning curve. Together they are a treasure trove of practical wisdom and smarts, but at first, they were not up with all the niceties of labor rules. Curiosity sometimes prevailed over legal prudence: "So are you planning on having children?" or "Why do you have that ball stuck in your tongue?" Good nursing homes prove that old hands can quickly learn new tricks of the cyber age.

Encouraged and supported by her Bethel Health Care family, Judson is always up to new tricks. One of her latest is a new program in which residents learn to become friends and partners who not only elevate the quality of their life but also add quality to their end-of-life experience. Their motto is at Bethel: no one dies alone. Therefore, the residents are mastering the meaningful touch and the hand-to-heart techniques of staying connected with a friend during the last moments of life.

CHAPTER 6

A Person-Centered Health Care Model

What a piece of work is a man, how noble in reason?
How infinite in faculty! In form and moving,
How express and admirable! In action, how
like an angel! In apprehension,
How like a god! The beauty of the world! The paragon of animals!
—*Hamlet*

This glorious paean to humankind was called into question on June 11, 2008. In a challenge to human exceptionalism, the autonomous region of Spain's Balearic Islands endorsed the Declaration on Great Apes (6.01).

The declaration extends the "community of equals" to nonhuman apes; it declares that they are entitled to the rights of life, liberty, and protection from torture. Apes may not be killed except under strictly defined circumstances, such as self-defense. They may not be imprisoned without due legal process, and they may not be subjected to the "deliberate infliction of severe pain," even if doing so is said to benefit others; they may not be kept for circuses, television commercials, or filming. Continuing to keep the 315 apes in Spanish zoos would not be illegal, but conditions would need to improve drastically in 70 percent of establishments to comply with the new law.

Animal protection has been a concern from ancient times. Hindus and Buddhists, in the third millennium before Christ, eschewed animal sacrifice, took to vegetarianism, and preached ahimsa. Notably, Emperor Ashoka (304–232 BCE) decreed against hunting and animal slaughter. At the same time, Greek philosophers and, later, Catholic theologians placed humans in the God-ordained chain of being. (6.02).

In recent times, many countries have recognized animal rights, but Spain, well-known for bullfighting, was a trailblazer in declaring nonhuman apes as moral persons with an inherent worth and dignity. It was a radical departure from the traditional concept of the unique human person. Soon, many countries, from Bolivia to Singapore, outlawed the use of some or all animals in circuses. New Zealand granted basic rights to five great ape species in 1999. Their use is now forbidden in research, testing, or teaching (6.03). Several European countries completely banned the use of great apes in animal testing. In 2010, Catalonia outlawed bullfighting, the first such ban in Spain. In 2002, Germany became the first European Union member to amend its constitution and guaranteed rights to animals (6.04).

This chapter offers a conceptual framework that puts the human person in context, makes meaningful its constituent elements. The human person, the cornerstone of humanistic health care, and the leitmotif of this book. For the purpose at hand, we skirt its philosophical ramifications, but we offer a social theoretical framework to understand the human person and human needs in the humanistic tradition and to evaluate how health care serves the human person's basic needs.

Part 1. The Human Person and Health Care

What, then, is the status of Shakespeare's godlike man? Who is a person? And what makes one a person? Much debate has swirled around these questions. The controversy has centered not only around animal rights but also groups of humans who have not always enjoyed human rights: women, slaves, minorities, and children. Humans have also wavered whether to accord such rights to extraterrestrial life and to legal entities such as corporations, estates, and other social constructs.

The public discussion has not led to a consensus on the exceptional elements that constitute a human person. However, among the important features that are commonly deemed unique to personhood are the following:

A human person

- has a sense of self, can be self-reflective, can self–evaluate;
- is rational, deliberate, hedonic, prudent, aesthetic, and ethical in making decisions;
- feels positive and negative sensations and emotions;
- controls own behavior;
- uses language, representations, and symbols;
- recognizes other persons and treats them as persons; and
- has a variety of sophisticated cognitive abilities.

The human person is pivotal to our discussion that takes guidance from the *Russell-Einstein Manifesto*, that set the lofty standard set in 1955: "Remember your humanity, and forget the rest" (6.05).

A Human-Needs Approach to Health Care

We view health care's obligations from a human-needs perspective. Chapter 5 discussed health care's social contract to promote human health and to cure illness. The question before us now is simple and direct. What do we expect from health care?

At the least, we expect that health care's policies and practices do not run counter to the goals of human life. Ideally, health care would be a catalyst to human well-being.

What is human well-being? What is the goal humans yearn for? Of course, the aim of human life is to be happy. But you cannot pursue happiness as a goal. You can experience happiness when you have achieved your life's goals—to stay alive, to be in good health, and to live a decent life with purpose and with meaning.

Humans do not choose these goals arbitrarily. Rather, they stem from needs deeply rooted in our nature. All humans yearn for the same goals because all share the same natural needs. The United Nation's Universal Declaration of Human Rights Article 25 states, "Everyone has the right to an adequate standard of living, including medical care and services, in sickness, disability, and old age."

Health care plays a sacred role as the satisfier of our natural need to stay alive, to feel safe, to cope with pain, and when ill, to be whole again. We judge how well health care lives up to its mission, in the compassion with which medicine promotes human health and healing.

Human Wants, Needs, and Rights

Humans have many wants and needs. Wants, desires, and aspirations range widely; they are not universal but specific to individuals. Human needs, as defined here, are those few longings that are present in all humans. They are natural or essential to all of us. They are not acquired or earned or conferred. They are built into the nature of human beings. They are part of what makes a rational person. The endow us our natural rights, make us valued as humans, confer on us the honor and dignity due to a person; they define our goals and drive our behavior.

Thus, all humans yearn to live and to avoid death, danger, pain, and illness. Every human seeks to be one's own self, to be respected, to be free, and to be able to control one's destiny. Every individual yearns to connect, to relate, to belong, and to be wanted. Every person wishes to rise to one's highest potential, to transcend themselves, act toward others with kindness and compassion, and thus add value, meaning, and purpose to their life.

A natural need begets a natural right—that is, it gives you a natural claim to fulfill your natural need. A natural human right imposes on society, on each of us, and on health care an obligation to acknowledge your claim.

We also have political, legal, social, and economic rights, among many others. These are, in effect, privileges conferred or curtailed by society or state. Their purpose is to ensure that we all live as good citizens and contribute to the collective quality of life. They are marginal to our purpose here, and so we give them marginal attention.

We draw on the rich tradition in humanism, especially on the needs-based themes. We observe the stalwarts amid us who have translated these themes into action plans to advance the cause of compassion. From this treasury of sources, we construct a concise model that that clarifies the goals of human life and health care's mandate to serve them.

Part 2. Five Core Human Needs

The human-needs perspective has been used in academia, in policy making, in economic and political analysis, in marketing, in product branding, etc. Various lists of human needs have been compiled and configured, varying in length, labels, and taxonomy.

The five needs that we consider as the core are a distilled formulation of what theory, research, and practice have established in the best humanistic tradition. These five needs are conceptually distinct from one another, but they overlap, interplay, combine, and configure in a multitude of patterns. They apply to various domains of human life. They are stated broadly here as a framework to clarify the complex developments in health care. As such, the template is open enough to accommodate new detail and nuance. It deserves a closer look and greater precision if it is to be validated through research.

A discussion on human needs cannot avoid a reference to Maslow (1908–1970). In his 1943 paper, "A Theory of Human Motivation," Abraham Maslow put out his now famous concept of the hierarchy of needs (6.06). He fleshed it out in 1954 in *Motivation and Personality*. Maslow studied "exemplary people" (Albert Einstein, Jane Addams, Eleanor Roosevelt, and Frederick Douglass) as well as the healthiest 1 percent of the college student population. His original list of five human needs grew into eight by 1970:

- Biological and physiological needs: air, food, drink, shelter, warmth, sex, sleep
- Safety needs: protection from elements, security, order, law, stability
- Love and belongingness needs: friendship, intimacy, affection, and love, from work group, family, friends, romantic relationships
- Cognitive needs: knowledge, meaning
- Aesthetic needs: appreciation and search for beauty, balance

- Self-actualization needs: realizing personal potential, self-fulfillment, seeking personal growth, and peak experiences
- Esteem needs: self-esteem, achievement, mastery, independence, status, dominance, prestige, managerial responsibility, form
- Transcendence needs: helping others to achieve self-actualization

Maslow Imitated and Modified: A Sample

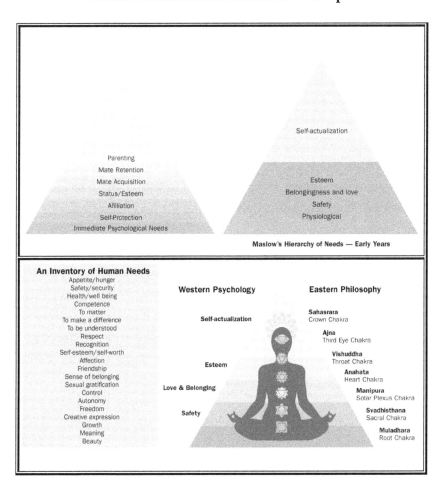

Parenting
Mate Retention
Mate Acquisition
Status/Esteem
Affiliation
Self-Protection
Immediate Psychological Needs

Self-actualization
Esteem
Belongingness and love
Safety
Physiological

Maslow's Hierarchy of Needs — Early Years

An Inventory of Human Needs
Appetite/hunger
Safety/security
Health/well being
Competence
To matter
To make a difference
To be understood
Respect
Recognition
Self-esteem/self-worth
Affection
Friendship
Sense of belonging
Sexual gratification
Control
Autonomy
Freedom
Creative expression
Growth
Meaning
Beauty

Western Psychology

Self-actualization

Esteem

Love & Belonging

Safety

Eastern Philosophy

Sahasrara
Crown Chakra

Ajna
Third Eye Chakra

Vishuddha
Throat Chakra

Anahata
Heart Chakra

Manipura
Solar Plexus Chakra

Svadhisthana
Sacral Chakra

Muladhara
Root Chakra

Maslow groups human needs in hierarchical structure; they are often portrayed in the form of a pyramid, although Maslow himself never depicted them in a pyramid. Just as some video games let you play at a higher level only after successfully completing the lower ones, the needs hierarchy requires that you fulfill the lower level of needs before you can satisfy those needs further up on the hierarchy.

Maslow's hierarchical model is widely adopted, imitated, modified, added to, and rearranged. It continues to be referenced in social psychological textbooks. But it has not held up well in many empirical tests. The theory of attachment in development has largely taken the place of Maslow's framework.

Maslow has been faulted for his flat and gross assumptions that are now seen as bound by time, place, and culture. Most seriously, Maslow talks about an individual's development in the absence of social connection and collaboration. "Without collaboration, there is no survival. It was not possible to defeat a Woolley Mammoth, build a secure structure, or care for children while hunting without a team effort. It's more true now than then. Our reliance on each other grows as societies became more complex, interconnected, and specialized. Connection is a prerequisite for survival, physically and emotionally" (6.07).

Other sophisticated needs-related models have generated intense academic and policy discussion. The Max-Neef model of human-scale development (6.08), Amartya Sen's model of human capabilities (6.09), and variations thereof by Martha Nussbaum (6.10) and others have dealt with poverty, justice, and economic development. They will not detain us since they do not shed light on the matter that concerns us.

The Human-Needs Perspective in Health Care

Many in health care have used the human-needs model to promote person-centered compassion in various areas in health care. They all affirm a person's right to decent health care. But each articulates and subscribes to a distinct mission, values, and agenda.

We offer here a thumbnail sketch of five such well-known examples of dedication to person-centered care in health care:

- The landmark report by IOM has been a springboard to launch innumerable programs.
- Picker Institute principles of patient-centered care led the field in formulating a framework for patient-directed advocacy.
- Planetree independently launched person-centered programs and emphasized the role of caregivers.
- The Pioneer Network has operated mostly in long-term care and served as a focal point for many scattered efforts at cultural transformation in long-term care.
- The Eden Alternative and the Greenhouse Project are specific organizational innovations that promote the primacy of human values in giving care to the elderly.

Across the Chasm: IOM's Six Aims for Changing the Health-Care System

In 1999, the Institute of Medicine (IOM) in Washington, DC, alarmed the public with its report *To Err Is Human: Building a Safer Health System* (6.11). The report drew attention to the crisis of patient safety in the delivery of care in the United States. IOM followed it up in 2001 with *Crossing the Quality Chasm: A New Health System for the*

21st Century (6.12). This report addressed the big gap in the United States between what good health care should be and the health care that people actually receive.

The report revealed a chasm separating what we expect of health care and what it actually delivers. It said that health care is fundamentally flawed and unable to reach the ideal. Real improvement calls for the whole system to change.

A restructured health care, IOM proposed, should have six aims. Health care should be as follows:

- Safe
  "First, do no harm" calls for accountability of individual practitioners.
  The IOM asks that health care assure safety in its clinical practice, procedures, and the delivery of care.
- Effective
  Health care should avoid underuse or overuse.
  Health care should be up-to-date and evidence-based.
- Patient-centered
  Treatment must address patient needs, preferences, and social and cultural links.
  The patient should be in control, have adequate information, be a partner in care, and be taught self-management.
- Timely
  Treatment should be prompt, information should be timely. Delay, if unavoidable, should not be discriminatory.
- Efficient
  Health care should avoid waste and reduce cost.
- Equitable
  Everyone should have access to health care regardless of race, gender, income, or education.
  State-of-the-art improvements should benefit all.

To achieve the six goals and thus to change health care root and branch, IOM advised that changes should occur at different levels:

- At the level of policy, payment, regulation, accreditation, and litigation
- In professional training, that shapes behavior, interests, and opportunities in health care
- In caregiving teams, their procedures, and their work environments
- In hospitals, clinics, and other health-care microsystems

The Joint Commission has energetically promoted these six aims. The IOM proposal, bold in its vision and radical in its prescriptions, prompted a defensive response from some but struck a chord in many. It has inspired many educational efforts and has resulted in many reformist activities, especially in hospitals.

It is clear that IOM's six aims are premised on the need and the right of all humans to have access to safe and humane treatment.

Picker Institute Principles of Patient-Centered Care

Harvey Picker had made his mark even before founding the Picker Institute. He had served as lieutenant commander in the U.S. Navy and had presided over and run Picker International (which manufactured x-ray, nuclear, and ultrasound imaging devices). At age fifty, he had gone to Harvard and Oxford, earned a PhD, and had become professor and dean at Columbia University.

The Picker Institute was founded in 1986 to promote a patient-centered approach to health care. Picker Institute Europe was established in 2000; by then, Picker Institutes were up and running in Sweden, Switzerland, and Germany. The Picker institute coined the phrase "patient-centered care"; it pioneered scientifically valid patient-satisfaction surveys for hospital patients. In 1993, it published the groundbreaking book *Through the Patient's Eyes: Understanding and Promoting Patient-Centered Care.* The book reflected the experience of a wide range of recently discharged patients, family members, physicians, and nonphysician hospital staff; it resulted in the identification of seven dimensions of care. These were renamed the Picker principles of patient-centered care in 1987. Access to care, an eighth principle, was added later. (National Research Corporation acquired from Picker Institute the rights to use Picker Surveys. In 2013, Picker Institute transferred its major programs to other institutions and ceased operations. National Research Corporation now owns the right to use the Picker Institute name and is continuing to develop tools and resources related to improving the patient experience under this name.)

The eight Picker Institute patient-centered principles are the following (6.13).

1. **Respect for patients' values, preferences, and expressed needs**
    Stay patient-focused; know the patient's medical needs and personal preferences. Provide information, give control, and teach self-management.
2. **Coordination and integration of care**
    Empathize with the patient's feeling vulnerable and powerless. Be sensitive to the patient's need for consistency and predictability.
3. **Information, communication, and education**
    Provide information on clinical status, progress, and prognosis. Give information on processes of care. Educate to facilitate autonomy, self-care, and health promotion.

4. **Physical comfort**

   Relieve and manage pain. Assist with needs of activities and daily living. Respect the patient's privacy. Keep areas clean and comfortable. Make the setting appropriate for visits by family and friends.

5. **Emotional support and alleviation of fear and anxiety**

   Relieve anxiety of the patient and family. Relieve anxiety over clinical status, treatment, and prognosis. Relieve anxiety over the financial impact of illness.

6. **Involvement of family and friends**

   Respect and recognize the family as patient advocate and decision maker. Support family members as caregivers. Recognize needs of family and friends.

7. **Transition and continuity**

   Provide clear information on medications, physical limitations, dietary needs, etc. Coordinate and plan ongoing treatment and services after discharge and ensure that patients and family understand this information. Provide information regarding access to clinical, social, physical, and financial support on a continuing basis.

8. **Access to care**

   Ensure patient's need to know how to access care when it is needed and about the time needed for admission and allocation to a bed. On ambulatory care, ensure the following:

   a. Access to the location of hospitals, clinics, and physician offices

   b. Availability of transportation

   c. Easy scheduling of appointments

   d. Availability of appointments when needed

   e. Access to specialists or specialty services when a referral is made

   f. Clear instructions on when and how to get referrals

The Picker principles were inspired by the IOM's aims and by what care receivers and caregivers told researchers in focus groups across the United States (6.14). They drew attention to the patient as a whole human person with emotions, family links, and cultural roots; they emphasized the just and dignified ways in which health care should address the needs of unwell humans. The theme is the humane treatment that we all deserve and to which we have a claim.

Planetree's Designation Criteria

Planetree was founded in 1978 by a patient to promote changes in health care that focus on healing and nurturing body, mind, and spirit (see Chapter 1). The first Planetree hospital opened in San Francisco in 1985. The thirteen-bed medical-surgical unit was planned and implemented in accordance with the wishes of patients, families, and health-care employees. The Planetree Network is now a global community of more than 250 hospitals, medical centers, continuing care communities, and rehabilitation centers in the United States and abroad. It establishes, at affiliate sites, a partnership of provider, patients, and families. It ensures good clinical care as well as comfort, dignity, and well-being of the patient. It creates a healing environment responsive to the well-being of patients and caregivers (6.15).

In 2007, Planetree pioneered the Patient-Centered Hospital Designation Program, the first to recognize hospitals with an operational infrastructure to sustain Planetree's culture of caregiving in its affiliate organization. Planetree has developed a criteria to determine if a patient-centered culture has been achieved.

In 2009, Planetree introduced a certification program for organizations that integrate the healing design into patient-centered caregiving. Its purpose is to promote a felicitous blend of the physical environment, architecture, and the culture of a caring community. It provides design professionals with a forum to understand the Planetree model of care and to give Planetree affiliates added resources to develop projects in a truly patient-centered model.

Planetree simply states that it believes the following:

- That we are human beings caring for other human beings.
- We are all caregivers.
- Caregiving is best achieved through kindness and compassion.
- Safe, accessible, high-quality care is fundamental to patient-centered care.
- In a holistic approach to meeting people's needs of body, mind, and spirit.
- Families, friends, and loved ones are vital to the healing process.
- Clear health information can empower individuals to participate in their health care.
- It is essential that individuals make personal choices related to their care.
- Physical environments can enhance healing, health, and well-being.
- Illness can be a transformational experience for patients, families, and caregivers.

Components of the Planetree Model

1. **Human Interactions/Independence, Dignity, and Choice**
   Human beings care for other human beings in a healing environment that gives personalized care to patients, residents, and their families and supports and nurtures staff. Planetree supports an individual's autonomy, lifestyle, and interests.

2. **Importance of Family, Friends, and Social Support**

The Care Partner Program encourages the presence and participation of family during admission, hospital stay, and discharge in the ICU and ER and during invasive procedures and resuscitation. It encourages families to stay overnight. It includes pet therapy.

3. **Patient/Resident Education and Community Access to Information**

Illness becomes a transformational experience. Patient charts are open; they can be read and commented upon. Patients participate in a self-medication program and learn self-management. Libraries and the Internet support self-care.

4. **Healing Environment: Architecture and Interior Design**

The physical environment incorporates healing, removes architectural barriers, encourages family visits and involvement, and provides space for solitude, prayer, and camaraderie or garden walks.

5. **Nutritional and Nurturing Aspects of Food**

Dining arrangements emphasize health and healing; they promote comfort and fellowship, encourage families to bring home-cooked food, and make kitchens available throughout the facility. Volunteers bake breads, muffins, and cookies; they provide aromatherapy.

6. **Arts Program/Meaningful Activities and Entertainment**

Planetree hosts classes, events, music, storytellers, clowns, and movies. Artwork in patient rooms, treatment areas, and residential spaces add to the ambiance. Art carts enable patients to select the artwork of their choice. Volunteers help patients and residents create their own art.

7. **Spirituality and Diversity**

Chapels, gardens, labyrinths, and meditation rooms provide opportunities for reflection and prayer. Chaplains are vital members of the health-care team

8. **Importance of Human Touch**
Training programs teach staff, family, and volunteers to learn hand and foot massages and offer internship programs for massage therapists.

9. **Integrative Therapies/Paths to Well-Being**
Aromatherapy, acupuncture, and Reiki offer options in addition to clinical care. To meet growing consumer demand for complementary therapies, Planetree has instituted heart disease reversal programs, guided imagery, therapeutic touch, acupuncture, Tai Chi, yoga, and aromatherapy. Exercise facilities are customized for seniors. Wellness programs focus on prevention and chronic disease management.

10. **Healthy Communities/Enhancement of Life's Journey**
Opportunities for wellness, personal growth, and self-expression include partnering with schools, senior citizen centers, and churches. Planetree chooses environmentally friendly cleaning products and sponsors kids' camps, walking clubs, and community gardens. Life stories programs capture milestones.

Planetree stands out as an inspiring accomplishment: it broke through the frontiers of biomedicine, expanded into different levels of care, broadened its scope of activity, and attracted an international following. And all this under the leadership of a foreign-born woman who heeded the promptings of compassion.

The Pioneer Network

Pioneer Network was formed in 1997 by advocates for culture change in all models of elder care and services, from long-term nursing home care to short-term transitional care and community-based care. Its goal is to create homes that are consumer-driven and resident-directed.

It envisions a culture of aging that is life-affirming, satisfying, humane, and meaningful. It supports models where elders live in open, diverse, caring communities. Its aim is to transform the culture of aging in America. Its stated mission is to encourage communication, networking, and learning opportunities (6.16).

It declares its values and principles are as follows:

- Know each person.
- Each person can and does make a difference.
- Relationships are the fundamental building blocks of a transformed culture.
- Respond to spirit, as well as mind and body.
- Risk taking is a normal part of life.
- Put person before task.
- All elders are entitled to self-determination wherever they live.
- Community is the antidote to institutionalization.
- Do unto others as you would have them do unto you.
- Promote the growth and development of all.
- Shape and use the potential of the environment in all its aspects: physical, organizational, and psycho/social/spiritual.
- Practice self-examination, searching for new creativity and opportunities for doing better.

- that culture change and transformation are not destinations but a journey—always a work in progress.

The Pioneer Network is a loose collection of individuals and without many organizational members. An ideological umbrella shelters a diversity of views, ideas, and ideals. Its conventions attract attendees in numbers that are envied by many. They attend less to learn than to share ideas for camaraderie and to regenerate one another.

The Eden Alternative

The Eden Alternative was founded in 1991 by William Thomas. It claims it has about two hundred registered members. Their aim is to create a life worth living for elders in their care. They encourage caring for other living things in a varied environment filled with plants, animals, and children. This model favors abandoning the traditional top-down bureaucratic approach to management and moving decision making closer to the elders (6.17).

The Eden Alternative summarizes its philosophy in the following statements:

- The three plagues of loneliness, helplessness, and boredom account for the bulk of suffering among our elders.
- An elder-centered community commits to creating a human habitat where life revolves around close and continuing contact with plants, animals, and children. These relationships provide the young and old alike with a pathway to a life worth living.
- Loving companionship is the antidote to loneliness. Elders deserve easy access to human and animal companionship.

- An elder-centered community creates opportunity to give as well as receive care. This is the antidote to helplessness.
- An elder-centered community imbues daily life with variety and spontaneity by creating an environment in which unexpected and unpredictable interactions and happenings can take place. This is the antidote to boredom.
- Meaningless activity corrodes the human spirit. The opportunity to do things that we find meaningful is essential to human health.
- Medical treatment should be the servant of genuine human caring, never its master.
- An elder-centered community honors its elders by deemphasizing top-down bureaucratic authority, seeking instead to place the maximum possible decision-making authority into the hands of the elders or into the hands of those closest to them.
- Creating an elder-centered community is a never-ending process. Human growth must never be separated from human life.
- Wise leadership is the lifeblood of any struggle against the three plagues. For it, there can be no substitute.

The Green House Project

The Green House Project grew out of the same philosophy. The first Green House Project home was constructed in 2003 in Tupelo, Mississippi. By 2014, there were more than two hundred such communities. It has worked primarily with providers of skilled-nursing care. Its principal distinction is a particular operational model to achieve person-centered care. It advocates care settings designed for ten to twelve residents, the comfort of private rooms and bathrooms, a family-like atmosphere, and open common spaces. It calls for self-managed teams of direct care staff working in cross-trained roles. Residents do not have strict schedules and are encouraged to interact with staff and other residents, families, and pets. Staff members and residents develop personal relationships with one another because of the small community and home atmosphere.

The Green House model is rooted in a philosophy of person-directed, relationship-based care. Those who live in or work in a Green House home foster late-life development within the daily life they create together. It sees elderhood as an opportunity for growth and development and is understood to have worth and meaning (6.18).

Part 3. An Integrated, Person-Centered Model

The five models we have summarized above approach caregiving within a human-needs perspective. They share the same goal but take parallel routes and overlapping strategy, each with its particular style and character.

A Comparison of the Five Field Models

Human-Needs Model		IOM: 6 Aims	Picker: 8 Principles	Planetree: 11 Criteria	Pioneer Network Beliefs	Eden/Green House Philosophy
5 Human Needs	**Need Components**					
TO BE						
· To be alive	Safety from injury, pain	✓	✓	✓		
· To be well	Primary care, public health, health education	✓	✓	✓		
· To be healed	Care: accessible, affordable, timely, coordinated		✓	✓	✓	✓
· To die in dignity	Dignity at end of life events		✓	✓	✓	
TO BECOME						
· To have self esteem	Care: wholistic, personal, respects privacy	✓	✓	✓	✓	
· To be in control	Consent, choice, control, self-manage-ment, being a partner	✓	✓	✓	✓	
TO BELONG						
· To bond	Connecting, empathizing, being compassionate		✓	✓	✓	✓
· To feel secure	Human warmth, relief from anx-iety and insecurity	✓	✓	✓	✓	✓
· To have comfort of family	Family involvement		✓	✓		
· To be connected	With community, children, pets, nature			✓	✓	✓

Human-Needs Model		IOM: 6 Aims	Picker: 8 Principles	Planetree: 11 Criteria	Pioneer Network Beliefs	Eden/Green House Philosophy
TO BE YOUR BEST						
· To grow as person	Making illness a teacher; learning new ways, lifestyle, and outlook	✓			✓	✓
· To strive, achieve	Know your strengths	✓	✓	✓	✓	✓
· To be a better person	Know your strengths, weakness, potential			✓	✓	
· To have meaning and purpose	Make pain and illness transformative			✓	✓	
TO REACH BEYOND						
· To transcend self	Minimize cost, avoid waste	✓				
· To empathize	Cooperate, comply				✓	✓
· To accept responsibility	Create joy, spread cheer			✓	✓	

Integrated Model: Assumptions

Our integrated model articulates the age-old sublime values and axioms of humanistic traditions, and its configuration draws on the person-centered programs that already successfully operated in the field. In short, we propose a model that takes the following as non-negotiable truths:

- Human life has intrinsic value and deserves our recognition, respect, and honor. It is primarily defined by the noble, higher human impulses, as exemplified by the very best among us: heroes, saints, and exemplars. Egotism, dominance, and exploitation are untamed prehuman residual tendencies; they are not what make us human.

- An individual is a whole person, indivisibly interconnected in body, mind, and spirit, and is shaped by a unique biography and life journey. Eternal vigilance is required as science and medicine disaggregate the person and risk dehumanizing us all.

- We are born to relate, to connect, and to lend a helping hand. The noblest form of human relationships is compassion: the awareness and acknowledgement of the suffering of another and the desire to relieve it. Altruism, which prompts us to put the interests of another before our own, often flows from compassion. Humanism envisions a health care in which an evidence-based approach guides caregiving, where an egalitarian, caring culture flattens hierarchy and promotes communication across gender, class, and rank divisions, where reason and humanity blend in nurturing a healing environment that caters to the needs of all participating in a health-care episode.

- We emphasize that the words *person* and *needs* do not apply only to the patient or resident; they embrace all participants in a health-care event: the patient and resident, the family, the caregiving team, and managers who set the supportive context. That is, whereas the patient with a physical ailment is the focus of attention, the care providers may also suffer from worries in their personal life, from needs unfulfilled and rights compromised. They yearn for solace and healing. They cannot bring wholeness to the patient if they are not whole persons themselves. Thus, a therapeutic event should occur within a healing context sensitive and responsive to the human deficits of patient and caregiver alike. A healing environment within a culture of caring is the ideal setting for person-centered health care.

In sum, the goal of life is to stay alive, to be well, and to live the good life. Wellness and a good life result when our basic needs are satisfied within a supportive community. When wellness is compromised, we look to health care to create a therapeutic setting that transforms suffering, gives meaning to illness, and makes us whole again.

Integrated Model: Components

A Human-Needs Model Turns a Care Setting into a Healing Environment

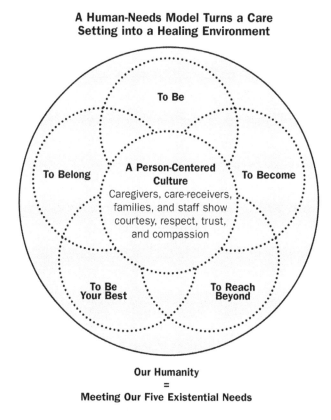

Our Humanity
=
Meeting Our Five Existential Needs

Five basic human needs are inborn and are natural to all humans in all human contexts: they are inborn and natural to caregivers in a therapeutic context. These needs give us our inalienable right to live and to live a good life. They are the following.

The Human Need and Right to Be

This need manifests as our instinct for survival, our lust for life. This need is primal and elementary—it precedes all other needs. We desire to avoid or postpone death so desperately that the ultimate punishment society metes out for a heinous crime is the death penalty. The ultimate self-sacrifice a martyr or jihadist makes on behalf of one's community is self-immolation. The final action a soldier takes to avoid surrender or an individual takes to avoid unbearable pain, disease, or humiliation is suicide.

The need to live makes us avoid risk of harm or injury and to adopt a lifestyle that promises good health—the foundation of well-being and a good life. When our health is compromised by sickness or pain, we turn to health care, expecting that our health will be restored and that we will be whole again.

Health care has an implicit pact with society (chapter 4) to help us stay healthy and to cure sickness. How well has health care fulfilled its pledge to serve our health-related needs?

Health care reform has to fulfill this basic human need by making hospitals and clinical treatment safe and free of risk. It has to assure all humans an easy access to health services and make them affordable. It has to actively promote health and well-being.

The Human Need and Right to Become

Everyone wants to be a unique person, to be recognized and respected for one's sake, to be valued intrinsically as a person. Everyone yearns to be free, to steer one's own life, to be in control of one's destiny, to be independent, and to live and die in dignity.

Does health care meet this need and right of a patient or resident to decide about one's care? To be fully informed, to learn self-care? Do customer preferences override institutional efficiencies when planning the daily schedule, meals, changing rooms, and transitions to and from the hospital? Is the care setting consonant with the dignity and privacy of life, dying, and death? Does it honor professional expertise, autonomy, and judgment of the caregiver?

The Human Need and Right to Belong

Humans seek to connect with family, friends, community, to the world, to nature. They want to be wanted and to belong. This longing is so deep-seated in humans that for ages, isolation has been used as a form of severe punishment. Research has firmly and overwhelming established that humans postpone death, guard against disease, and enjoy greater satisfaction in life when they relate to people in a bond of marriage or friendship.

How does health care fulfill its obligations in this regard when technological medicine and disengaged clinical professionalism frown upon familiarity, affiliation, and the caring touch? An emotionally sterile professionalism starves out compassion, makes treatment less satisfying, clogs communication, diffuses accountability, erodes trust, and thus sets the stage for errors to occur and to go unreported, for patients to be harmed, and malpractice suits to soar.

The Human Need and Right to Be Your Best

Humans crave not only to exist but also to live and to enjoy a full life. Context, time, and circumstance may keep us fenced in and may even thwart our yearnings, but we still thirst to grow, to create, and to bring to flower our talent and skills. Self-actualization seeks to close the gap between what we are and what we could become.

Health care has not fully embraced its calling as a teacher. The biomedical slant in health care has discounted the existential aspects of pain, suffering, and illness. Medicine has dealt with pain and sickness as physiological dysfunctions; it has paid scant heed to the redemptive meaning that can turn pain into a spiritual awakening and make sickness open a window to self-knowledge, new possibilities, and a new direction to life.

The Human Need and Right to Reach Beyond

This need, the most virtuous and illustrious of human urges, compels us to rise above selfish promptings and to give ourselves to others. It refers to the virtue of altruism, cognate to empathy and compassion. Empathy makes us look at the world through the eyes of another; compassion takes us into the personal world of the other and makes us share the pain and to cosuffer.

Altruism is a call to generosity, to serve and to give unselfishly. In their most sublime form, these virtues blend and find expression in a person who gives generously, knowing fully that the recipient is unable to reciprocate. Humans have a need to self-transcend. We relish the inner reward when we rise above egotism and self-absorption, as does a mother, a friend or a healer.

Our natural urge to transcend reinforces the solemn responsibility each of us bears to others for the privilege of being human. It engages us in a cause larger than ourselves; it adds value to our life, gives us a purpose to live a meaningful life.

Patients and residents are not merely recipients of care; they bear a responsibility to the needs of their family, to the caregivers, and to society—to all who have a role when we are ill. The care receiver has to be sensitive and responsive to their needs and, thus, to contribute to the healing of all.

Abundant evidence attests to the spiritual and health benefits that flow from altruism. The evidence does not support the "survival of the fittest" view. Rather, research findings validate the truth of survival of the kindest, in evolution, in life, and in health care.

In sum, modern medicine has chalked up a splendid record; it helps extend human life span, it rescues us from fatal trauma, from deadly infection and from crippling pain. That achievement has been clouded by health care's legacy of error, injury and lack of heart. How do we judge how well medicine has lived up to its Hippocratic Oath and up to its social contract? An answer raises the paramount question: Who is the human person that health care is obligated to serve? What are the basic needs that give every human person the inalienable right to expect that health care to respect and to satisfy them? We have identified five human yearnings; we flesh them out in the following chapters and hold up health care efforts to meet them.

CHAPTER 7

The Human Need and Right to Be

We are going to die, and that makes us the lucky ones.
Most people are never going to die because they are never going
to be born. The potential people who could have been here in
my place but who will in fact never see the light of day outnumber the sand grains of Sahara. Certainly, those unborn ghosts
include greater poets than Keats, scientists greater than Newton.
We know this because the set of possible people allowed by
our DNA so massively outnumbers the set of actual people.
In the teeth of these stupefying odds, it is you and I, in our ordi-
nariness that are here. We privileged few, who won the lottery of
birth against all odds, how dare we whine at our inevitable return
to that prior state, from which the vast majority has never stirred.
—*Richard Dawkins*

To Be Alive, to Be Safe, and to Be Well

It is nothing short of miraculous that you won the lottery of birth.
Countless eggs are washed away from every mother's womb. Millions
of sperm are released in one ejaculation. And just one egg got fertilized by one sperm in one split second and became human, and that is

you. You won against the one-in-billions odds. Then you won again when most of the fertilized eggs got aborted without the mother knowing it; you survived. The meeting of one particular sperm with one particular egg and the particular biography of one woman's pregnancy gave you your personal identity.

Leading British evolutionist Richard Dawkins, in his autobiography, *An Appetite for Wonder* (7.01), asked, "What if Alois Schiklgruber had sneezed at a particular moment in the years before mid 1888 when his son Adolf Hitler was born?" Dawkins feels certain that a sneeze would have been sufficient to alter history. Out of the billions of sperm Herr Schicklgruber produced in his life, that one evil-omened sperm could have been derailed and not met that particular fateful egg that engendered Adolf Hitler.

Indeed, Dawkins has wondered if we mammals owe our existence to a particular sneeze by a particular dinosaur. In other words, the lottery of birth begins much before conception. What are the odds that your parents met and gave birth to you? What is the probability that your parents came into the world? And so the odds increase astronomically as we look in the rearview mirror way into the past, where we see the dinosaur sneeze. What are the odds that in the wide universe that mother earth was picked at random and that random events converged and nurtured life?

In this dazzling panorama of life, we humans are less than a speck of dust, but each of us is specially blessed. We are here despite all odds. To be alive as humans is doubly lucky. We are also privileged to be aware of our habitat, to appreciate its grandeur, and to make a graceful exit, leaving behind a better world than we found.

Great souls have reflected on the sacred truth of human life:

We grow up; but the world remains a child.
Star and flower, in silence, watch us go.
And sometimes we appear to be the final
exam they must succeed on. And they do.
—*Rainer Maria Rilke*

The nitrogen in our DNA, the calcium in our
teeth, the iron in our blood, the carbon in our
apple pies were made in the interiors of collaps-
ing stars. We are made of star stuff.
—*Carl Sagan*

Part 1. The Culture of Life

This chapter discusses the sacredness of life, our obligation to support one another in preserving and enhancing life, and health care's
mandate to rescue, to safeguard, and to prolong life. We will point
to health care's notable efforts to prolong life, to banish pain, and
to hasten recovery. We ask how health care's safety record compares
with what aviation has done to make air travel safe. Finally, we examine how broadly health care applies the notion of the human person
and, specifically, how well it takes care of its own, how much it values
the life of the direct, frontline caregiver.

The primal hunger for life, deeply etched into the human DNA,
has been a principal concern of every society. Every major religion has
upheld the sacredness of human life. The Catholic Church has felicitously labeled its reverence for life as a "culture of life" (7.02). The
United Nations has echoed the consensus of 171 nations that the
"inherent dignity and the equal and inalienable rights of all members
of the human family is the foundation of freedom, justice and peace
in the world… All human beings are born free and equal in dignity

and rights. Everyone has the right to a standard of living… including food, clothing, housing, and medical care… and the right to security in the event of unemployment, sickness, disability" (7.03).

Our inalienable natural right to life obligates each of us to recognize, respect, and value all human life. It also charges each nation-state with an obligation to honor life, to institute ways to improve the life of its citizens, to protect them from harm, and to mend and heal when their health is compromised. This natural right constitutes a mandate for health democracy. That is, the state has to ensure that everyone has a fair and equal access to health care, and care providers should respect the humanity and dignity of life whatever the condition of the patient.

Has Medicine Delivered on Its Promise?

One area where medicine has earned high praise for meeting its obligations is by answering its call to protect life and to cure it when needed is that it has harnessed medical research, knowledge, and technology to combat the most dreaded enemies of humanity—sickness, pain, and death. Doctors routinely reconstruct mangled bodies, redesign brains with bullet holes, conduct surgery in utero, and fight off mysterious new infections emerging out of unexplored hot zones. *U.S. News and World Report* (July 15, 2014) reviewed the medical advances of the last twenty-five years and featured a handful that have saved lives, extended our life span, and added quality to life (7.04, 7.05). Health care has dramatically cut mortality rates, has lessened the risk of surgery-related infection, has made serious surgery minimally invasive, has made surgery less painful and recovery faster, has made a quicker return to work possible.

Treatment and surgery today are safer and less painful (appendix A details the recent clinical innovations that have brought dramatic benefits to patients).

Health care has advanced in another front.

In the 1990s, several countries revealed the hitherto hidden problem of patient injuries and deaths. In the United States, the Institute of Medicine's 1999 report *To Err Is Human: Building a Safer Health System* (7.06) led to the Patient Safety and Quality Improvement Act of 2005 (Public Law 109-41) to be signed into law on July 29, 2005 (7.07). It was a response to the goal of the act to improve patient safety by encouraging the reporting of adverse events. Both government and private safety-promoting organizations soon came into being, dedicated to improve health-care safety: error reporting, research, education, training, and dissemination of best practices—they are generically referred to as patient safety organizations (PSOs) (see Appendix B). PSOs, foundations, and interest groups and from the World Health Organization hold retreats, give workshops, and conduct seminars and teach-ins. They teach, they motivate, and they offer practical tips.

Health care has lived up to its obligation to make medicine safe by devising tools and processes to avoid risk. The following are a representative of these types of innovations.

- Simple feedback practices. Commonsensical redundancy pays high safety dividends. Lucian Leape explained, "You call your favorite Chinese restaurant and order your favorite dishes. Before you hang up, the restaurant person says, 'Let me read your order back to you.'" This simple, highly effective read-back practice can forestall a lapse when a doctor phones in a critical order, but it was not hospital policy anywhere until The Joint Commission mandated the read back of patients' names and oral orders (7.08).

- Open-notes practice is followed at Harvard and Beth Israel Hospital in Boston and at Kiesinger Medical Center in Pennsylvania. It gives patients online access to their doctors' notes. Some physicians read back their notes on patient history and diagnosis back to the patient and ask patients to provide editorial comments and corrections.

- Standardized communication is indispensable. Surgeons now initial the surgical sites to make sure they don't cut off the wrong leg. Before The Joint Commission regulated the practice, some surgeons marked the site on their own. Some put an *X* on the leg to be operated on, and others put an *X* on the leg not to be operated on.

- Debriefing sessions improve patient safety. A weekly gathering of doctors, nurses, and other personnel (off-limits to the public) engages in a candid, no finger-pointing discussion of mistakes, complications, deaths, and unusual cases. Doctors hold one another accountable and learn from one another's mistakes. A 2012 study found that debriefing in a hospital OR, done consistently, soon after a procedure and for the express purpose of identifying systemic issues identified 6,202 defects concerning instrumentation, radiology, laboratory, supply, and communication and safety in forty-four months. (7.09)

- A daily safety huddle of key leaders, now used by many hospitals, came directly from a practice used on aircraft carriers. At Cincinnati Children's Hospital Medical Center in Ohio, "Every morning at 8:35 a.m., departments all have to report on three things: what happened that didn't go quite right, what are the risks I'm managing for the next twenty-four hours, and what's broken or needs to be fixed?" said Stephen Muething, vice president for safety (7.10).

- Computerized provider order entry (CPOE) systems greatly reduce order transmission errors. Checklists are used in various clinical procedures. Devices with radio frequency keep track of surgical tools and blood-soaked surgical sponges. A software warns doctors when patients' prescriptions interact badly.

- Making rooms exactly similar and equipment arranged in exactly the same place prevent accidents. Prominent door signs as part of protocol prevent infections. It is much easier to avoid errors if the environment has been designed to avoid them, but this hasn't been so in health care. The architectural landscape is changing according to Ellen Taylor, director of research at the Center for Health Design. Guidelines for new construction of hospitals and outpatient facilities require a safety risk assessment, for example, determining whether nurses can see a patient from the nursing station or standardizing in each hospital room the location of equipment such as medical gas outlets, disinfectant gels, and used needle containers.

- WellStar Paulding Hospital in Hiram, Georgia, situated sinks so patients can see handwashing. It uses soap dispensers that monitor handwashing via a wireless system that identifies staff who do not comply. It eliminated thresholds to step over, situated the head of the bed less than a yard away from the bathroom door, and installed a handrail and night-light between them. Its patient rooms accommodate family members who function as observers of care. Patients, friends, and family are increasingly seen as key strands of the safety net.

- Artemis March collated for the Agency for Healthcare Research and Quality (AHRQ) "Stories of Success: Using CUSP to Improve Safety." They are accounts of how four hospitals applied a patient safety model called the Comprehensive Unit-based Safety Program, or CUSP, to dramatically reduce central line-associated bloodstream infections (CLABSIs) and other health care–associated infections (HAIs). The cases address the origins of each facility's journey to eliminate HAIs, the organizational processes put into place, how CUSP champions overcame resistance and promoted ownership and accountability, and how CUSP is being sustained in units and spread into other areas of the hospital. One story demonstrates how easily CUSP was integrated with another quality-improvement method. Intensive care units, for example, are known to be dangerous places because they're packed with devices such as medication infusion pumps and ventilators that don't align with each other or with the patient's electronic medical record. One of those "little things" happened when an ICU nurse made a drug error because the small vial packaging print was very difficult to read. The hospital put magnifying glasses all over the ICU (7.11).

- Karen Curtiss wrote *Safe & Sound in the Hospital* after her father had a successful lung transplant but died following a series of subsequent medical errors. The book offers checklists for preventing infections, blood clots, bed sores, and other common complications (7.12).

- Julia Hallisy became a safety advocate after witnessing a variety of errors, including a delayed sepsis diagnosis, during her daughter's ten-year, ultimately fatal struggle with retinoblastoma. "I started to write down all the things I wanted to be sure we remembered," recalled Hallisy. "My daughter asked what it was, and I said 'I'm writing down all the things we've learned about keeping you safe.' She said it should be a book." The eventual result, *The*

Empowered Patient Hospital Guide for Patients and Families, is crammed with practical advice, such as asking a pharmacist to be directly involved in your treatment if you have a complex drug regimen (7.13).

- In 2004, 125 Michigan ICUs took part in a project to prevent deadly CLABSIs using CUSP. Bloodstream infection rates fell by 66 percent in these Michigan hospitals. In 2008, 1,100 hospital teams in adult ICUs in forty-six states used CUSP and have reduced the rate of CLABSIs by 40 percent, saving more than five hundred lives and avoiding more than $34 million in health-care expenses (7.14).

- The Department of Health and Human Services said in May 2014 that hospital-acquired complications fell 9 percent between 2010 and 2012, from 145 to 132 per one thousand discharges. The Centers for Disease Control and Prevention reported in 2014 a 44 percent decrease in central line bloodstream infections between 2008 and 2012 (7.15).

- Cincinnati Children's has seen an 80 percent reduction in serious patient safety events since 2006 and is aiming for zero by the end of 2015 (7.16). Bronson Methodist Hospital, in Kalamazoo, Michigan, saw a 45 percent drop in hospital-acquired infections in units that had done away with semiprivate rooms (7.17).

- At Bassett Medical Center in Cooperstown, New York, staffers' compliance with hand hygiene rules has shot up by nearly a third since patients began receiving a document called "Partnership for Patient Safety," which ticks off ways they can help protect themselves. The document states that staffers are supposed to wash their hands when they come in and check each patient's wrist ID upon entering the room, when giving medications and drawing blood, and before leaving for any procedures, for example. If these precautions aren't followed, patients are encouraged to ask (7.18).

- In Tennessee, a ten-hospital collaborative reduced complications and saved $2.2 million per one hundred cases and saw a significant reduction in site infections, according to a study published in 2012 in the *Journal of the American College of Surgeons* (7.19).

- The nonprofit Leapfrog Group, focused on improving hospital quality and safety funded by employers that purchase health care, found in a 2014 survey that almost one-third of hospitals have seen a 10 percent or higher improvement in their performance since 2012 on a host of measures, including hand hygiene and giving proper antibiotics before surgery (7.20).

- Some precautionary interventions can be programmed into the system. Thanks to an inspiration of some medical residents at New York-Presbyterian Hospital, electronic health records now prompt staff to take the crucial step of comparing patients' medications to what they're being given in the hospital. A hard stop prevents further medical orders from being executed if the task hasn't been completed within eighteen hours of admission (7.21).

Part 2. Human Error in Health Care and Aviation

Health-care innovations seem to have handsomely contributed to human health. In order to put these gains in perspective, it is instructive to compare health care's achievements in patient safety to the safety record of aviation. In aviation, passenger safety is as pivotal as the motto "First, do no harm" is in health care.

Humans like to speed on ground and in air; they have paid a hefty price for trying to speed ever faster. Airplanes, trains, trucks, buses, and ships—complex machines—do much harm. Globally, traffic crashes kill 3,500 people each day, including 720 children. That is, traffic accidents kill 1 million people and injure about 50 million annually (7.22).

The world's first aviation accident occurred on September 17, 1908. Orville Wright had lengthened the previously proven propeller design by four inches. This untested propeller struck the other propeller; the aircraft pitched and took a fatal plunge. This mishap prompted a search for safety. In the early phase, aviation focused on improving technical, engineering causes of risk. Although the accidents in the air began to fall, they remained high for the next twenty-five years.

On October 30, 1935, test pilot Les Tower joined Major Ployer Peter Hill who, as Boeing's most experienced test pilot, had test flown sixty of the Army Air Corps' newest aircraft. It was a competition between Martin-Douglass Aircraft and Boeing Model 299—the future Boeing B-17 Flying Fortress, the first plane with four engines that could fly twice the range, 30 percent faster, with five times the payload (7.23).

The two took off from Wright Field in Dayton, Ohio. At three hundred feet, the plane stalled, crashed, and killed the two men.

The cause of the crash? The pilot forgot to release the tail elevators. People said it was just too much airplane for one man to fly. Complexity was not the cause; Boeing did not need a redesign. It introduced a checklist. The B-17 and its checklist flew the next 1.8 million miles without an accident. The military purchased over thirteen thousand, and the B-17 was the workhorse of the Allied air force in World War II.

Weather systems, metal fatigue, incorrect radar data, mechanical flaws, failing electrical systems, tainted fuel, and hydraulic failure cause accidents. Injury results from ill-designed concourses and jet ways, slippery and ill-lit floors, food poisoning, and terrorist acts. But human error causes over half of all aircraft-related injuries. Errors occur wherever humans are involved, whether it is pilots, crew, workers who fuel, those who do maintenance, conduct inspections, or handle baggage.

In a span of twenty years, from 1938 to 1968, the aviation fatality rate fell tenfold, as low as the state of technology would permit. In the second phase, aviation concentrated in guiding human behavior along the nonrisk path. It took another thirty years for the fatality rate to decline another tenfold. During these thirty years, risk managers wrestled with the task of changing organizational behavior to turn workers into partners with a shared goal of maximizing safety. Today, the aviation industry's compliance to high standards is routine in most regions of the globe. In the United States, 137 airlines out of 448 have a top seven-star rating.

In 1946, eighty-three accidents per one hundred thousand flying hours were recorded. By the mid-1950s, accidents declined to ten per one hundred thousand hours. For the recent fifteen years, they have plateaued and have hovered around 1.25 to 1.75. Commercial aviation has had zero fatalities for the past few years (7.24).

Chesley Sullenberger, the hero of the Miracle on the Hudson, said, "The risk of accidental death in a jet aircraft from 1967 to 1976 was one in 2 million. Today, it is one in 10 million. After 75 years, we in aviation have benefited from lessons learned at great cost—literally bought in blood—lessons we now offer up to the medical field for the taking."

Dr. Arnold Barnett, MIT flight safety expert, calculated that over the fifteen years between 1975 and 1994, the death risk per flight was one in seven million. If you flew every day of your life, it would take you nineteen thousand years before you would succumb to a fatal accident (7.25).

Aviation's Pursuit of Safety: Lessons for Health Care

American aviation falls into four categories:

1. Military aviation owned by the government
2. Civilian scheduled Commercial Aviation (CCA) with domestic and international operations
3. Civilian General Aviation (CGA), regional commuter passenger air service to communities without sufficient demand to attract mainline airlines
4. Civilian General Aviation (GA), noncommuter ranging from gliders and powered parachutes to fire-fighting, agriculture-related, and corporate jets

CCA carried 2.9 billion passengers in 2012 and 3.1 billion passengers in 2013. GA flights take off from 5,200 airports in the United States and over 1,000 in Canada. CGA regional flights operate from around 560 airports in the United States and serve about 50 percent of all air passengers (7.26).

In its pursuit of patient safety, health care has chalked an impressive string of victories. Many of them have occurred in hospital settings. Hospitals have resorted to ways—use of simple tools to installation of elaborate systems.

Health care as a vast and varied field outmatches aviation in complexity. There are 13,000 known diseases, syndromes, and injuries; 4,000 possible tests; 6,000 medications, treatments, and surgeries; 5,722 hospitals, 700,000 active physicians, and 2,600,000 active nurses; they write 3,899,799,770 prescriptions a year. A generalist physician receives more than 3,500 annual visits, while a specialist receives around 2,700 visits. As treatments and procedures multiply, the possibility of error increases, and the urgency of systems-based reform becomes imperative.

The epidemiology of aircraft accidents offers a valuable lesson on the notion of systems and on the philosophy and policy that have made aviation the exemplar of safety.

The CCA outshines GA in performance and safety outcomes (7.27):

- GA noncommuter aircraft have an accident rate six times higher than the CGA regional commuter airlines and forty times higher than the CCA commercial air transport.
- Over the past ten years, GA noncommuter aircraft increased their accident rate by 20 percent and have held a steady 6.8 injuries per one hundred thousand flight hours, while CCA decreased accidents by more than 80 percent and fatality by 25 percent.
- Annually, GA noncommuter aircraft have 1,500 accidents and more than 400 fatalities among pilots and passengers.

CCA and GA share many features; they follow similar rules and use similar equipment. The difference in their performance is pronounced and persistent, and for good reason. CCA and GA noncommuter airlines are worlds apart in character, purpose, and practice.

GA noncommuter:

- Operations are predominantly single pilot.
- Range of operations is wider and riskier: aerial taxi, banner towing, law enforcement, firefighting, and crop dusting.

- Aircrafts are smaller, have fewer cockpit resources and different purposes and motivation.
- Pilot training and qualifications greatly vary regarding difficult weather and new technology.
- As a group, they are less cohesive, monitored less stringently and unevenly.
- Pilots bear responsibility for safety not shared with dispatcher or meteorologist.
- Uses thousands of landing facilities; many lack precision approaches, long runways, and good lighting.
- Has more takeoffs and landings per hour—the highest-risk phases of a flight.

Aviation's Systems Approach

Small operators frequently transport their families and friends. Fatigue, medical condition, poor sleep, family tension, and alcohol can impair cognition and compromise safety. In contrast, GA operations have more built-in inherent controls and can draw on extensive support.

Aviation's safety record is the envy of health care, which has borrowed heavily from aviation. However, realistically, we should not expect the imports from aviation will help health care take a giant step toward safety. In the insightful words of Rishi Sikka, senior vice president of clinical transformation at Advocate Health Care, a 250-site health system based in Downers Grove, Illinois, "A lot of folks who look at safety focus on the things we need to do with nurses and physicians, but none of that works on the frontline if culture and leadership aren't there" (7.28).

Systems, culture, leadership, and in the context of health care, compassion—these are the ingredients in aviation's success. They are the sine qua nons of any meaningful reform in health care. After the initial novelty wears off, an imported practice will wilt if not grafted on to integrated systems and not nourished by a culture of mutual caring under a compassionate leader.

System refers to a planned interaction between discrete parts that are linked to, interdependent on, and interacting with on another; all parts work toward a common goal. At the beginning of the twentieth century, Émile Durkheim referred to a social fact (values, norms, and structures) that exists outside of individuals. Like a system, it is a force unto itself; it can drive and shape behavior of individuals within the system and without (7.29).

Edward Deming, whom the Japanese venerate as a quality guru for turning their postwar industry around, descended on Detroit in the early 1980s at the behest of Ford CEO Donald Petersen. Ford was hemorrhaging red ink and was battered by Japanese competition. Deming introduced the U.S. industry to the statistical method that gave us the six sigma measures of quality.

Aviation Safety in Perspective

In 2013:
- Three billion people boarded 35 million airline flights.
- Each of them travelled over 500 miles per hour, in an aluminum tube, seven miles above the earth.
- Zero people died.

In 2013:
- Falling out of bed caused over 400 deaths and 1.8 million emergency room visits.
- Vending machines toppled and killed 13 people.
- Over 300 people drowned in bathtubs.
- Texting while driving killed 6,000.
- Hippos killed 2,900 people.

Deming dinned into the auto moguls in Detroit the fundamental principle in sociology: good systems are critical to the success of any organization (7.30). Managers create systems that guide performance and affect the quality of the outcomes. Deming maintained that 80 percent of quality problems in any enterprise, and in health care especially, should be laid at the door of the managers. Systems dictate behavior. Good workers in bad systems produce bad outcomes. Structures, policies, and workplace culture all act as systems that transcend the individual.

CCA has a big lesson to teach health care. CCA committed itself early to the goal of risk avoidance and to safety management systems (SMSs). It partnered with international organizations. It put its personnel through training and learning programs. It rallied member airlines to embrace the cause of safety. In its first phase of ensuring passenger safety, it introduced technical innovation and cut accidents tenfold. It repeated that feat in the second phase by reducing risk caused by human error. In its third phase, it pursued safety on the organizational level. It partnered with international bodies, like the International Civil Aviation Organization (ICAO). Together they have vigorously pushed airlines to avoid risk by adopting safety management systems. In its current phase, aviation's thrust is on the cultural level with the aim to erect a bulwark against risk, namely, a just culture of safety.

SMSs rest on assumptions and principles of humanistic sociology, anthropology, psychology, and management, although SMS manuals do not dwell on its philosophical origins. These principles are the core of the safety projects ICAO designs to train airlines about SMSs. As an airline becomes more immune to risk, the more SMS takes firm root and matures into a culture of safety.

Aviation's goal is a just culture of safety built on humanistic principles—the most important lesson it has to teach health care. Its approach rests on the following assumptions:

- A just safety culture encourages trust, transparency, and self-disclosure of error.
- It builds a consensus on what is acceptable and nonacceptable risk.
- It puts error into three groups: an inappropriate but inadvertent slip, an uninformed mistake, and a conscious disregard of grave risk.
- A just safety culture consoles those who inadvertently slip. It educates and trains those who are short on prudence or skill. It deals firmly but humanely with those who err because of reckless risk taking.
- It is a fair culture. It rewards responsibility and accountability. It values learning over punishment. It turns error into a learning experience.

- A just culture does not incriminate or point fingers. It makes self-reporting of error an expectation and a virtue.
- A flexible culture lets you bend rules but not their spirit or intent.
- Absence of accidents is not absence of risk. Risky behaviors may not have led to accidents by simple luck. SMSs anticipate the possible and stand ready and alert for challenges unknown.

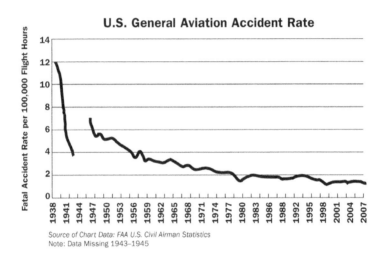

U.S. General Aviation Accident Rate

Source of Chart Data: FAA U.S. Civil Airman Statistics
Note: Data Missing 1943–1945

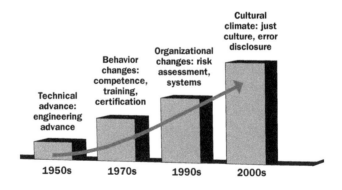

Aviation's Progress Toward Safety: Four Phases

Safety Flows Downwards

- Top managers are the foundation of SMS. Compassionate managers lift a risk-prone hospital from the ashes and infuse it with a just SMS culture. An exemplary health-care organization can quickly flame out when a good administrator leaves and a mediocre one takes the place.
- Managers make workers partners in a shared mission.
- Good managers do not rely only on rewards and sanctions. They trust, delegate, and give workers room to grow. They make workers feel vested in the organization. As true partners, they share goals, strategy budgetary, and other information with the workers.

"Many, many hospitals have hired pilots to do team training and crew resource management. We closed the ORs, did these 'rah-rah' sessions and nothing changed. What worked for aviation teamwork is not necessarily going to work for health-care teamwork," says Dr. Pronovost, one of many who bemoan the problem (7.31).

The Pronovost diagnosis falls short of the mark. Why have safety-promoting tools floundered in health care when they have proved effective in aviation? Some imports from aviation have succeeded in isolated pockets; most have withered.

Just as the human body rejects surgical implants, so do established cultures look askance at attempts to introduce alien ways and mores. Most hospitals unwittingly foster an amoral culture, which in turn will not take kindly to new behaviors that run against the grain of long-established interests, values, and habits.

Safety and Error Reporting in a Trusting and Caring Workplace

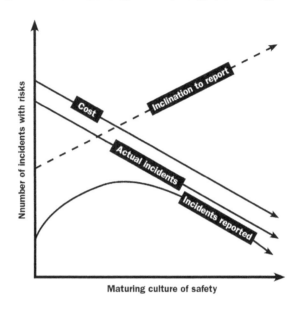

The Checklist: Promise and Reality

A case in point is the now-famous checklist that originated in the cockpit but has been hailed as a shortcut treatment for health care's woes.

The word *checklist* invokes the image of a simple-minded tool. In fact, an aviation checklist is a sophisticated product whose design requires a significant investment of brain work, experience, and research.

In *The Checklist Manifesto*, Dr. Atul Gawande describes the WHO study that he directed in eight cities around the world with diverse economies and patient populations: Seattle (USA), Toronto (Canada), London (England), Auckland (Australia), Amman (Jordan), Ifakara (Tanzania), and New Delhi (India) (7.32). From 2007 to 2008, surgical teams at these eight sites participated in the WHO's Safe Surgery Saves Lives program. They used a used a two-minute, nineteen-step checklist during operations on 3,955 patients.

The rate of any complication at all sites dropped 57 percent, and the in-hospital rate of death dropped 87 percent. Rates of complication at high-income sites fell 31 percent and 39 percent among lower-income sites. The rate of death was reduced 3 percent at high-income sites and 52 percent at lower-income sites. WHO, sponsor of the study, estimated that at least five hundred thousand deaths per year could be prevented through worldwide implementation of this checklist.

Its worldwide fame led to its widespread adoption. The United Kingdom implemented a nationwide program within weeks after the checklist results were published in the NEJM. Almost six thousand hospitals worldwide are actively using or are on the way to implementing the checklist (7.33).

Then, amid the checklist jubilation, the rough-and-tumble realty of health care set in. Checklist implementation tripped on a fact of life familiar to researchers. Researchers conduct experiments in a lab-like setting stripped of intervening distractions. Their valid findings, when implemented, often falter and stall in the contradictions and compromises of daily practice.

A Canadian study assessed the success of the surgical checklist in 133 surgical hospitals in Ontario, a Canadian province with a population of more than thirteen million people. The Ministry of Health and Long-Term Care had mandated public reporting of the outcomes of surgical safety checklists for hospitals beginning in July 2010. The hospitals were, on their own, implementing the required surgical safety checklists in Ontario—an excellent setting to evaluate the effectiveness of checklist use.

"We couldn't identify a measurable improvement with checklists," said lead researcher Dr. David Urbach, a professor of surgery and health policy at the University of Toronto. Either singly or cumulatively, the hospitals showed no benefit in the use of checklists (7.34).

Communication failures are common in surgical care; they lead to errors and patient harm. Communication failures in the OR occur in 30 percent of team exchanges, and a third of these jeopardize patient safety (7.35). The checklist stresses the importance of communication based on an egalitarian, open exchange communication across hierarchy, rank, and gender.

By that logic, unless the ongoing checklist practice is infused into the bloodstream of a hospital's day-to-day culture, it will regress into a sham ritual. Like any other import, a checklist will strike root and prosper only in a compatible host culture.

Unfortunately, too many hospitals will find this an insurmountable task. Life in a typical hospital runs by the protocols of hierarchy. Formalities of rank and privilege undermine trust and sharing, which are highly prized in the checklist context. Self-disclosure of error, the heart of a just culture of safety, runs counter to legal caution and to the intent of the Fifth Amendment. In fact, reporting one's error is tantamount to self-incrimination; a nonblaming safety culture turns error into a teacher and reporting it a virtue. It rewards accountability.

The checklist protocol prescribes a presurgical checklist huddle meant to introduce the surgical team members to one another; it serves as a token substitute when a hospital lacks a friendly tie among and across departments and disciplines. Gawande found some of the countries that participated in his eight-nation study had gender- or status-based hierarchical cultures. The social inequalities of everyday life carry over into the surgical room with deleterious effect on communication. However, success of the checklist approach depends on equal relationships and teamwork. Thus, in hospitals where friendly exchange was common, preoperative checklist huddles did not show significant positive outcomes, presumably because they were super-fluous (7.36).

Scot Ellner, coauthor of the study "Communication Failures in the Operating Room" says, prior to surgery, "Introductions are crit-ical. As the surgeon, I think it's important for members of the team to address me by my first name, and we make sure that everyone else knows each other by their first name. Calling someone by his or her first name elicits trust. In the operating room you want to feel comfortable with your team and know that they will respond appro-priately during the most challenging cases" (7.37).

The culture of a typical hospital is a bastion of social status, rank, and privilege. Imagine this scenario. A new young female nurse, Elvira, is assigned to OR duty where the checklist protocol is being implemented. The checklist instructs Elvira that she is an equal member of the team. It calls upon her to be sure to raise the alert, to stop, or to report an inadvertent serious error she may happen to notice, like the one the chief surgeon is about to make. Do we really expect that Elvira has what it takes to live up to that mandate? To override the rules of gender and rank that she has learned through life and has been reinforced by the hospital culture?

When a hospital's policies, priorities, and practices do not favor these egalitarian values, we should not expect that innovations like the checklists and The Joint Commission's Universal Protocol to yield substantive, long-term positive outcomes.

Part 3. To Live and Be Well in Long-Term Care

Person-centeredness, we have argued, enjoins that we respect the life and humanity of the caregiver as much as of the care receiver. In one of our interviews with a surgeon, we brought up the case of a (fictional) doctor, emotionally disturbed, psychologically impaired, and in search of spiritual redemption. Did the surgeon know of such cases? Yes, many more than he could count. "What help do such struggling doctors seek or count on?" we asked.

"There is always the hotline," he deadpanned.

How about long-term care? How does health care as a profession care for its own? Here, we ask, How well does health care safeguard caregivers from harm and make them feel secure?

Caring in a Harsh Workplace

Safety is of paramount concern for elders in a nursing home. But critics allege that residents suffering abuse occurs in nursing homes. Abuse, indeed, is common in nursing homes, but it is directed mostly against caregivers.

CNAs are the backbone of long-term care, the largest direct caregiver group. More than one in two of us will spend some time in a nursing home; one in four of us will die in a nursing home. CNAs will minister to us in our last days on earth. The well-being and goodwill of the CNAs will determine the quality of our life during those last days and hours.

Many residents, families, and visitors verbally and physically assault CNAs. Some residents with an intact mind and a sharp tongue verbally abuse, hurl racial epithets, humiliate, and provoke their caregivers. Some mean-spirited residents, for all we know, were mean, uncouth, and racist in their younger years; they have grown into old age uncleansed and unredeemed. They find an easy target in CNAs. Residents with dementia (about 60 percent) on occasion discharge a volley of creative insults at them.

CNAs are routinely accused of everything from stealing dentures to gross physical abuse. Even when innocent, a CNA pays an undeserved price. Regulation requires that the accused be investigated. The CNA is presumed guilty and bears the burden of proof. Many CNAs have told us that at deposition and when testifying, trial lawyers expose to the world the CNA's dark side that she had not suspected was a part of her makeup. It is a pitiable contest: a vain glorious lawyer versus a thoroughly shaken CNA. Bear in mind that 75 percent of CNAs have only a high school diploma, while 12 percent do not possess a high school diploma or GED certificate. When the ordeal ends, the scars and stigma linger; they strain friendships and affect the aide's career (7.38).

In 2010, Dr. Helena Miranda studied nursing homes in Maryland and Maine and found that residents and visitors routinely attack CNAs and other caregivers. In a three-month period, residents and visitors had attacked half of the caregivers at least once; a quarter of the caregivers were attacked repeatedly (7.39).

The nursing home, the prison, and the mental asylum are settings where clients turn violently on those who serve them. But unlike the other two sites, a nursing home does not routinely train CNAs to deal with difficult residents and visitors. One CNA wrote this open comment: "Patients don't have a 'right' to physically hit you, but I've been punched, kicked, spat upon, and pinched in an inappropriate place by a dementia patient. Combative patients are not easy to work with but require patience and 'extra care' and time to manage them. I had one skinny ninety-year-old patient who could summon the strength and fighting spirit of a warrior. I needed a second person to help care for her."

Caregiving: A Backbreaking Job

To the risk of harm from others, add the risk of working in a backbreaking workplace. As direct caregivers, CNAs help residents with the activities of daily living, such as bathing, eating, dressing, and toileting. They, more than anyone else, lift and reposition residents, who in recent times come from the hospital sicker and more physically dependent. Lifting and repositioning residents in bed or transferring them in and out of the bed or chair turns out to be a backbreaking job.

Using proper body mechanics may not prevent injury, because lifting adult patients is intrinsically unsafe. Lifting becomes more dangerous when the resident is bigger, heavier, uncooperative, and combative; the room is small and cluttered; and the bathroom entry and layout are inconvenient. When the bed prevents bending the knees, as happens all the time, and the CNA bends forward, she puts her spine in a very vulnerable position. Even under ideal conditions, an adult far exceeds the lifting capacity of most CNAs as 92 percent of them are women, and 12.5 percent are fifty-four years or older (7.40).

A 2012 research paper on 1,500 nursing homes reported what caregivers suffer when serving seniors:

- The 2011 Bureau of Labor Statistics data shows that workers in nursing and residential care facilities now have the highest injury rates of any occupational setting. This is a move up from third place five years earlier (behind construction workers and truck drivers).
- Of the three-quarters of a million CNAs in the fifteen thousand nursing homes, 60.2 percent report a workplace injury a year, with 8 percent of these injured more than once. The injured CNAs averaged 4.5 injuries per CNA. Almost 16 percent of injured CNAs were limited to lighter work, while 25 percent badly injured CNAs missed three days of work on an average.
- CNAs report scratches, open wounds, and cuts (45 percent of injured CNAs); back injuries (18 percent); black eyes

and bruises (16 percent); strained muscles other than back strain (16 percent); human bites (12 percent); and other injuries from blows, kicks, being punched, grabbed, run over, and bumped into (7 percent). A substantial number of the injuries (like black eyes and human bites) indicate aggressive encounters with residents, families, and visitors.

- Most CNAs (87.6 percent) reported that lifting devices are always available, and 10.3 percent reported that they are sometimes available. Only a few CNAs reported lack of access to assistive equipment. Whether a CNA uses lifting devices and how much does not depend on whether the devices are available or whether the CNAs have been oriented to use them. It depends on how much managers care about them as people, shield them from abuse, and create a safe workplace.

Who will care for our caregivers?

We end this chapter summing up the principal conclusions we are left with. Medicine has lived up to its promise in one important regard. It has beaten back our dread enemies—disease, pain, and death. But many innovations to promote person-centered care, including the imports from aviation, have wilted, withered, or are in danger of dying on the vine. They are transplants unwelcome in a cultural climate conducive to biomedical values than supportive of the humane ways of compassion.

Health care's shortcomings are, in the final analysis, a failure of leadership. The cornerstone of health-care quality is the manager. Leaders in medicine at best stood by and at worst allied with outside forces, steering clinical training and practice away from its compassionate origins. Only enlightened, wise, and compassionate leaders can steer the health care ship toward that compassionate safe harbor. The rank and file in health care, with a supportive public behind them, will have to devise ways to screen, select, and recruit such leaders starting at the very top.

A clear agenda awaits such leaders. It calls for a redesign of systems and structures so they give primacy to the human person, i.e., they support true professionalism of practitioners; they make caregivers and staff partners in governance; and they invite patients, residents, and families to be partners in caregiving. An established culture will only yield to a compelling, humane agenda led by a bold, compassionate leader.

Models and Exemplars: How Ordinary Women Do Extraordinary Things
V. Tellis-Nayak, PhD

Note: *The authors studied these indefatigable women, the very exemplars of compassion, who meet the primal need of the poorest of the poor to stay alive and to be safe. The place lies far across the seas. Its message speaks to the whole wide world.*

Nicholas Kristof of *The New York Times* travels to hidden corners of the globe and chronicles the incredible feats of the human spirit. In remote lands, he has seen Catholic nuns defy warlords, pimps, and bandits. They are, he says, the bravest, toughest, and most admirable people in the world.

I too have an edifying nuns' story. It began a hundred years ago in a neighborhood I know well. It continues to unfold to this day with undiminished vigor. To show you heroic nuns in action, let me take you to a special corner of the world, Mangalore, India, where I was born and grew up. Mangalore and its culture are the backdrop for my story.

A coastal town on the Arabian Sea, Mangalore's considerable charm is fast yielding to the untidy, unsightly, and unseemly ravages of modernity. Christians walked in my neighborhood in India much earlier than they first walked the streets of Paris. St. (Doubting) Thomas, apostle of Jesus, first brought Christianity to this shore a bit south of where I lived; Vasco da Gama ushered in Western Christianity a bit farther south. Today, Christians are India's third-largest religious group; they outnumber Christians in many European nations. Although they are a mere 2.3 percent of India, Christians make up 30 percent of Mangalore's population; they are mostly Catholics who have created a distinctive Mangalore Catholic culture, which has nurtured countless nuns and priests.

Among the foreign missionary nuns and priests that streamed into town were three Sisters of Charity from Italy. They arrived in Mangalore on January 24, 1898, and set up a hub just a stone's throw from my family home. As an altar boy, I served Mass in the Chapel of Maria Bambina, which the three Sisters built at the entrance to what has developed into an incredible operation—the fruit of the nuns' mission of charity.

In an area less than two square blocks, the Sisters of Charity today house and minister to hundreds of society's rejects—from young orphans to very old elders and many others in between, broken in body or in mind. Some of them staggered up to the convent door. The nuns found some others dying on the roadside. They brought home newborns abandoned by impoverished mothers and the mentally disturbed wandering the streets. The nuns took them in because they all met one criterion: they were utterly destitute. Sister Sylvia, the nun in charge, is called upon every day to affirm her mission—she says no to successful or well-off people who go to her and offer generous donations if the nuns could take in their live-alone aging parent. They do not qualify by the sacred priorities of the nuns.

The Improbable and the Implausible

The buildings sit along the outer perimeter of a central courtyard. The Infant Mary Convent houses fifteen professed nuns and five student nuns. The extension to the convent, the infirmary, accommodates ten nuns who seem as old as the hills and have labored countless years in the Lord's vineyard. The younger sisters minister to them in their frail, ripe years. Other buildings house 185 elderly, 100 mentally compromised persons of all ages, and 107 youngsters (most of them orphans) and a few boarders enrolled at the school across the walkway run by the nuns. The living environment is clean and offers minimal creature comforts, adequate by local standards but an upgrade from the dire condition from where most residents came.

The numbers seem improbable. Five of the nuns, together with lay helpers, administer and teach at the high school. Some nuns serve or study at places outside the campus. That leaves just six nuns to assume total responsibility for the lives and welfare of three-hundred-plus disparate individuals whom society has bypassed.

Here's another incredible detail. These indefatigable women hire no staff except for two commuting women who serve as volunteer workers. Yes, there are few other workers who help in the kitchen, in caregiving, or wherever else they are needed. Their formal schooling is meager. What skills they have were learned under two mentors: life and experience. The workers expect no remuneration because the nuns cannot afford to hire them for pay. They are content to live with those whom they look after, to share their meals, and to walk in the nuns' footsteps.

Many such unconventional practices add to the mystery of this implausible nuns' story.

Mother Theresa, My Neighbor

The nuns move with grace from the sacred to the secular, and vice versa, as they blend a life of prayer with the call of charity. They don't miss community prayers or meals and find time for daily personal meditation and prayer. They are always busy in an unhurried way. They get up long before the sun rises and are still on their feet hours after it sets. Weekdays differ little from weekends. The calendar shows no scheduled vacations, mental-health days, or personal days. Occasionally, they go on a picnic, a train trip a couple of hours due east, to bond with their fellow nuns engaged in similar work. They celebrate feasts and festivals with style and verve, with song, dance, and laughter.

Their ways are mundane, their days lack excitement, and their life has no glamour. But the ready smile on their face and the subtle spring in their step bespeak of minds at peace and hearts touched by joy. The witness they bear wins admirers and wide support; it draws volunteers and inspires young women to follow their footsteps.

If this story seems to you to be just a variation on the story of the fabled nun Mother Theresa, you are exactly right. Mother Theresa was indeed an exceptional soul, but she was not an exception. There are many Mother Theresas—countless women tirelessly pushing just causes in never-ending struggles that would have defeated lesser mortals. They are not just a lighter version of Mother Theresa. They are no less Olympian in moral stature and no less selfless in dedication than the legendary nun. Their most endearing trait is genuine humility—a mark of greatness; they avoid the spotlight, hide their achievement under a humdrum lifestyle, and live as your average next-door neighbor. So talent scouts do not discover them, they do not make the headlines; they do not win a Nobel Prize.

But you cannot ignore the light of their shining example that stirs the better angels within us.

A Simple Way to a Lofty Goal

It is a warm January evening in my hometown, Mangalore, India. My wife, Mary, and I are in a fervent dialogue with Sister Sylvia, the head of the Sisters of Charity, Infant Mary Convent. We stroll under a majestic canopy of towering coconut trees toward where the young beneficiaries reside. Hugs, kisses, and handshakes greet us. Inside, over a hundred pairs of eyes bulging with curiosity await us. At the cue from the stern matron, our miniature hosts erupt in a thunderous welcome in Kannada, the native language.

Without any cue, Mary rises to the occasion. First, she regales the tots with a couple of Yankee hits and then leads them in song-and-dance routine, instantly winning friends.

We make the rounds; we observe, question, and listen as the nuns' story plays out before us in living detail. Much of it uplifts and inspires. We find things that baffle and others that make us sad.

Mending Broken Lives

Residents across all groups revere the nuns as angels incarnate and not only because of all that the nuns have done for them but principally because of how the nuns connect with them. To the nuns, their charges are not patients, clients, or objects of charity. The nuns know each one by name, and they relate to them, across the status barrier, as humans, each deserving the dignity and honor due a person. First, they rescued them from a brutish world. Ever since, they have sheltered, fed, and clothed them. The nuns do not always cure their physical ailments, but they sure can heal a fractured soul, to make one feel like a person worthy of respect.

You cannot but be impressed by the power and potential of the nuns' caring touch and how deftly they use it to soothe a troubled teen, to make the newly admitted and thoroughly shaken widow feel at home, and to add some comfort and joy to the last moments of a dying man.

You cannot but be amazed that the nuns have restored life, humanity, and laughter to thousands of pathetic specimens of humanity, shunned as society's dregs. They have done this so consistently, so continuously, and with such dedication for so many years that the Mangalore community applauded the Sisters of Charity in a public ovation in 2012, the one hundredth year of their exemplary life.

Moreover, Sisters of Charity repeat this feat in varied formats in forty other locations in their state in India. Their example and their spirit of charity have beckoned generations of young Mangalore women to seek happiness through selflessness and transcendence.

These nuns put social scientists in a spot. Their everyday heroism defies easy explanation. By any measure, the Sisters of Charity come out as outliers.

Unsophisticated Ways

Their success, however, results from no outlandish method or arcane formula. Their approach, simple and unsophisticated, may strike a Western professional as naive. The complex operation is not built on a secure financial foundation. The nuns have no significant cash reserves, no endowments, grants, or subsidies. They do not conduct campaigns and capital drives. This fiscal insecurity aligns with their religious vow of poverty and does not disturb their equanimity. Theirs is an implausible world, where the improbable does not surprise you. Donations come in, mostly in kind. Here, residents have never gone hungry or been ill-clothed.

The nuns lag behind in one regard, and they know it. "We should do better in the clinical area," a nun admitted. They have no medical director and no physician on call. A physician drops by on occasion, but the nuns cannot afford to buy the medicines. So they take full advantage of the health-related camps sponsored by the Lions Club, the Rotarians, medical schools, open-air clinics that offer checkups, conduct surgeries, dispense drugs, etc.

We had expected the nuns to be more familiar with the material props that aid their spiritual mission. We did not find recent innovative tools, techniques, protocols, and best practices pertaining to assessment and care planning. Sadly, this leads, for example, to overuse of physical restraints when dealing with combative or unruly behavior.

Their training as nuns exhorted them on virtues of charity, self-abnegation, and humble service. What they learned about health care is inadequate for the challenge they face. Among those directly engaged with the residents, Sister Sylvia is a trained and experienced pharmacist, and Sister Alphonsa in psychiatric nursing, but she is only partly involved in this venture. The campus has no nurses or nurse assistants. The residents come from dire settings and may have more than their share of health problems. Thus, with no adequate professional help, they soon learn to be interdependent, to give mutual care, and to assume a brother-help-brother role.

In the Company of Heroes and Saints

We pondered over our experience, searching for links to care in the United States. We were thoroughly surprised that many of us in the United States who labor in long-term care share a kinship with Mother Theresas in faraway lands. Abroad, across the great divide, battered by wind and wave, we are driven by a common goal in the service of others.

At every turn, you find that the world is unfair and unequal; it shunts the weak and the unlucky to the margins; it creates an unequal system, deeply entrenched and self-perpetuating. Laws of the jungle prevail over the Ten Commandments. But deprivation cannot shackle the indomitable human spirit. In my hometown, it finds expression in the heroic women who strive to restore life, love, and joy to the victims of the world's sins.

Extraordinary deeds are not uncommon in nursing homes in the United States, which are so vastly different from Mangalore. Nursing homes get a bum rap. The reigning stereotype sees nursing home staff as untrained, uncommitted, and unloving. Regulators assault their professionalism, and oppressive rules dampen their best instincts. Yet hundreds of thousands of CNAs tell us (in satisfaction surveys), year after year, that the greatest satisfaction they get working in a nursing home is knowing the difference they make in the life of the elders. Conversely, hundreds of thousands of residents in those very nursing homes also tell us that among all their experiences of nursing home life, they are most satisfied with the care, concern, and respect they receive from their caregivers.

So we are, after all, fellow travelers with heroes and saints. We live in different worlds but need one another. Health care in the United States has a few things to teach Mother Theresas around the world—a greater openness to science, adoption of innovations in nursing, and adapting the best practices, tools, and methods of the digital age.

But health care in the United States has raced too fast and too far down the road of technology and specialization. Giant progress in technology has robbed health care of the caring touch and has turned it cold and impersonal. Many stalwarts are trying to restore humanity and compassion to health care. In this monumental task, we can seek inspiration and guidance from the Mangalore nuns, the champion healers of the soul.

CHAPTER 8

The Human Need and Right to Become

And the day came
When the risk to remain tight in a bud,
Was more painful than the risk it took to blossom.
—*Anais Nin*

"Come to the edge."
"We can't. We're afraid."
"Come to the edge."
"We can't. We will fall.'
"Come to the edge."
And they came.
And he pushed them.
And they flew.
—*Christopher Logue*

Hunger for life is the first of the five inherent urges that define us as humans. The second is the urge to be yourself, to be someone distinctly you. Being the best is great; it makes you number one. Being unique is greater; it makes you the only one. Every person yearns for a unique distinct identity, to be the author of one's destiny, to be fully informed and to make one's own choices. These needs are our rights that make us valuable for our own sake and worthy of honor and dignity. A person elicits respect and recognition intrinsically, not derivatively.

A shared humanity makes us invaluable. We are all equal because each of us is worth the same, and each of us is priceless. However, equality is not commonality; equality does not make us same. You and I are equal yet profoundly different. We are, each one of us, an original. "Every one of us is precious in the cosmic perspective," says Carl Sagan. "If a human disagrees with you, let him live. In a hundred billion galaxies, you will not find another."

Dr. Seuss assures us that there are no duplicates of you or me in circulation:

> Today you are YOU,
> That is truer than true.
> There is no one alive
> Who is Youer than You.

We are unique at two levels. First, each of us is a blend of stardust mixed in different measures and cultured in different settings. Second, each of us has navigated life through sunshine and sorrow, we have triumphed sometimes, and we have stumbled often. Through toil and travail, we have become what we are today—each a unique biography and a distinctive identity.

Chapter 6 outlined how these basic human needs are at the core of the mission of modern medicine. This chapter looks at this second layer of foundation on which our humanity rests. We ask how our desire to be unique and autonomous plays out in the health-care arena,

In the preceding chapters, our argument drew heavily on the hospital world. In this, we focus more on long-term care. We will dwell on how the human need to become our own self sharpens with age, how the human spirit runs the gauntlet set up by old age, and how good managers help residents and caregivers to take control of their own life and destiny.

Part 1. Aging and Self-Worth

Our wish to be respected for our own sake, to be recognized as free, independent, and unique persons, becomes more urgent and salient as we advance in age. The case of Marge Donovan, one of our ideal types from chapter 2, illustrates what caregivers know. Symbols of independence become ever more important as age makes us increasingly dependent. Self-worth is an essential aspect of our self-image.

The most trying hardship of old age is not the unwelcome change to which aging subjects our body but how that change affects us as persons. Aging gives the signal for the body to begin to fall apart. As your body depreciates, you lose your ability to see, hear, speak, and taste. Age clouds beautiful minds; it dulls the best talent and blunts skills honed over a lifetime. Aging tests your spirit and resilience.

Worse, the slow-motion demolition of your personal and social life reverberates through every fiber and pore. Aging spares nothing and is hardest on your self-concept. Dependency devalues you and your self-worth. You are still the matriarch but with no pedestal. You pick up the unintended clues; your family is looking for a nursing home for you. It hurts, deeply.

Now your mind reviews dreaded scenarios. The anticipated move to the nursing home will not be just a change in residence; rather, that move will uproot you from the ecosystem that you painstakingly put together over the years and which has become your social skin—soft, congenial, and reassuring. The innocent laughter of children will no longer regale you. The move will dismantle your emotional supports. It will take away your informal and unfailing network of vigilant neighbors, loyal friends, professional colleagues, and spiritual mentors and guides. Your familiar, self-sufficient, and secure world collapses around you, just when you need it most. Instead, you are on the way to the nursing home, where you will spend the final days of life in the company of strangers and an endless flow of unfamiliar faces.

This inglorious fall from grace pushes you to the edge of the dark pit of depression.

Symbols of Dependency

Just like Mrs. Donovan, many dread going to a nursing home. Even the most caring nursing home worker does not wish to end up in a nursing home. A nursing home symbolically proclaims to the world the bitter truth: people do not find your craggy looks attractive or your company interesting, and you are of not much use to the world. That blow to your ego is too much to bear. When you feel you are less than a person and life has lost meaning, you look for an exit. Some elderly attempt suicide when faced with admission to a nursing home (8.01).

Old age poses a special challenge to health care. The ravages of age stymie your innate quest for individuality, recognition, and respect that make you a unique person. Thus, aging is more than a mere fact of life; it is also a symbol of diminished humanity. So a nursing home becomes a public symbol of human frailty and dependency.

The Resilient Spirit

What becomes of those who end up in the nursing home, reluctant, discouraged, and depressed though they may be? An answer to this question refers us to a subject that seldom shows up on the biomedical radar screen, namely, the resilience of the human spirit and its undying quest for happiness by fulfilling inherent human needs.

Suicide statistics illuminate this issue. The just over one hundred suicides a year in the nation's fifteen thousand nursing homes are lower (fifteen per one hundred thousand) than suicides for elders in the general population (sixteen per one hundred thousand). More people die by suicide than homicide. Suicide rate increases with age. Fourteen older adults (aged sixty and up) kill themselves each day. Older adults make up 14 percent of the U.S. population but account for over 16 percent of all suicides. Death rates by suicide reach their peak among the eighty-five or older group (twenty-eight per one hundred thousand) (8.02).

These numbers point to two conclusions. First, old age is a hard phase of life. The suicide rate spikes at sixty-five and is the highest among the very old. Second, nursing homes protect many elderly from self-inflicted death. Many go to nursing homes kicking and screaming, some are survivors of attempted suicide, some are shaken, and some are depressed. These and other factors put residents at risk. Yet nursing homes have a lower suicide rate than the elderly living in the community. Besides, almost half of deaths by suicide in nursing homes occur in the six months after admission (8.03).

Other findings fill in the picture. The multitude of satisfaction surveys in nursing homes, whether conducted in-house, by third-party vendors, universities, or researchers, all show consistent results on key issues across types of surveys and over the years. MIV by National Research Corporation, the biggest player, has used scientifically constructed survey tools over thirteen years in four-thousand-plus nursing homes. It has built an archive of structured and open-ended responses from nursing home residents, families, and staff. An independent assessment of responses from these three groups shows corroboration and consistency. And their overall judgment is consistent with what state surveyors say about the quality of care in those respective nursing homes (8.04).

In each group, upwards of 40 percent rate their satisfaction as excellent, and about 2 percent as poor. They would recommend their nursing home to others as a good place to receive care or as a workplace in even more positive numbers. Each group rated eighteen areas of nursing home life. Two areas consistently earn the highest satisfaction grade from residents and families: they feel safe, and the staff shows them respect and treats residents with concern.

These findings run contrary to the negative image of a nursing home in the public mind. They also show that the inhumane nursing home residents in the minds of new admits is now seen by them as their home. This is tribute indeed to the caregivers as well to the resilient and indomitable human spirit.

As the body ages and wilts, the human spirit does not necessarily atrophy or languish. Our primal need to be recognized may go unfed. Our right to be autonomous and free may be trampled upon. But the primal urge adapts and finds enclaves of happiness. Darwin's maxim is at play here. He said, "It is not the strongest of the species that survives, or the most intelligent, but the one most responsive to change." Mrs. Donovan exemplifies the truth of this dictum. When she could not cling on to the make-believe world of independence, she mounted a pouty, noncooperative protest and kept it up for three weeks. She knew its futility, but Mrs. Donovan had to affirm her self-esteem. She decided she had made her point, and that was adequate satisfaction. So she quietly swallowed her pride, faced reality, and blended in with flow of life in the nursing home. She found it fun.

Some have alleged that nursing home life responds more to the demands of institutional efficiency than to the residents' need for individuality and choice. Nursing homes too quickly get new residents to conform, comply, and thereby deprive them of autonomy and control. They see Mrs. Donovan's case as surrender. They do not recognize the silent victory of human ingenuity. Our survival instinct has taught us well; when we cannot control the wind, we need to adjust our sails. Letting the best be the enemy of the good is not a good survival strategy. Many elderly know well that in life, you do not get what you deserve but what you negotiate.

Part 2. Managers, Work, and Self-Identity

Barbara Dempsey and Dawn Sylvester are two nurses in their late forties. Barbara has worked in the same hospital for most of her career and risen very high in the estimation of her colleagues. She has refused time and again the offer to move into management. Her joy comes from caring for postoperative patients.

Dawn is a clinician of the first order, competent, bright, and likable. She has worked for companies large and small, giving direct care and in supervisory positions. She has won commendation in both roles. They do not come better than Dawn.

Barbara and Dawn are located in two distant corners in the Midwest. They do not know each other, nor have they heard of each other. But both were in the pool of nurses we interviewed repeatedly and at length. We talked with them separately about their part in the pledge health care has made to society to promote our health and well-being.

Health care's pact with society entrusts the nine million caregivers and other health-care workers with a sacred obligation to meet the health needs of those seeking help. That healing encounter between the health-care worker and the patient is the litmus test of health-care quality, whether it occurs in the hospital, the nursing home, or at the insurance or Medicaid office. Compassion's triumphs come from the two-way care and concern between the patient and the care-givers like Barbara and Dawn.

A compassionate encounter is the natural fruit of a humane culture, which in turn is the handiwork of a manager concerned about the well-being of the worker. Their varied experiences have led Barbara and Dawn to an identical conclusion: health-care quality rises or falls by the humanity a manager displays toward the caregiver.

Barbara provided a stunning illustration. A group of venture capitalists saw her hospital as ripe for the plucking; they brought about a merger and put in place new management. They announced an immediate reengineering of the hospital. The director of nursing was the first casualty. They added her duties to those of the DON in the other merged hospital twenty-nine miles away. The new CFO reset the productivity quotas and goals. Barbara and her fellow nurses saw themselves reduced to a cost item. The marketplace lingo and efficiencies ruled the day. Productivity became the new buzzword, and the hospital now measured it by the hour and logged it scrupulously. Nurses kept an eye on the clock as they cared for the postsurgical patients. And they did this for a good reason: if the census fell during the day, they sent nurses home in the middle of a shift and counted the lost hours of work as part of the nurses' personal and sick days; they counted a delay over three minutes to show up at work as delinquency punishable with dismissal. Morale hit the cellar. "You don't see any smiles in our hospital," says Barbara.

Dawn too worked in a dehumanizing setting and had to find a new employer, and she did. She now works for a company run by managers who are the very exemplars of person-centered concern for the workers, to whom we will refer below. Her previous employer was a large, for-profit chain of nursing homes that sought to diversify its holdings and acquired the regional outfit Dawn worked for. The chain had a mediocre reputation, but still, Dawn was shocked at their slash-and-burn strategy, seemingly meant to please Wall Street—the source of their venture capital.

Workers on three twelve-hour shifts who were deemed to put in a forty-hour workweek learned that their thirty-six actual hours of work fell short of the new definition of full-time work; that made them ineligible for overtime compensation and benefits that accrue to full employment. The company's pharmacy switched to generic medicines. They billed food supplements as extras and used them widely. Low-end, generic-brand clinical and personal-need supplies appeared on the shelves.

A Profile in Compassion

In the humanistic tradition, the measure of a good health care manager is not the ROI at the quarter's end but the commitment the manager evokes in the workers. A manager earns worker loyalty by relating to workers as unique persons, respecting them as individuals, appreciating their talent, empowering them, and setting the stage for them to succeed. The quality of the care a patient receives depends on how successfully the manager has turned the worker into a devoted caregiver.

We referred to the exemplary managers Dawn works for now. We studied several such luminaries in long-term care. One of the brightest stars in that firmament is Jayne Clairmont, a sharp entrepreneur with a compassionate instinct, a leader with a vision, and a jolly companion anyone would love to call a friend.

After college, Jayne worked for a long-term care firm, where the owner became her teacher. She listened carefully, watched intently, and learned much about how not to manage and how not to treat employees. That lesson learned, she went looking for a place to put her management skills to the test.

She scouted around residential neighborhoods in Minneapolis. She found a stately looking vintage house. With no ready access to capital or a family fortune and unwilling to go begging on Wall Street, Jayne frequented estate auctions and clearance and bankruptcy sales. She used the acquisitions from her treasure hunt to gussy up the home with an elegant touch. Along with a partner, she hung out the shingle English Rose Suites and set up shop. She canvassed for six dementia-care residents to live family-style in the elegant home, under the care of young women Jayne handpicked and personally trained.

Her concept was simple but timely; it preceded by a decade other costly versions of mini nursing homes. It struck a chord. In no time, English Rose Suites reached 100 percent occupancy. But trouble came from an unexpected corner. A cantankerous neighbor worked himself into a frenzy alleging that the mentally ill living on his block would depreciate the value of his house. In court, he inflated his case and alleged that Ms. Clairmont was engaged in a clandestine sex trade. That cheap shot boomeranged; two of Jane's residents were retired justices in the Minnesota courts. Now Jane runs five such homes in similar surroundings with less testy neighbors.

Jane says that her proudest accomplishment is the building of a well-knit team that serves the dementia residents with excellence and devotion. She reserves a special corner of her heart for her staff. Jayne recruited each of them for their skill, talent, and potential to be part of the caring English Rose Suites community. She delegates and thus shapes the next generation of leaders. She is fully engaged in recruiting them, teaching them the nuances of dementia care, and keeping them abreast of the latest developments in their field. She assigns books to read, she takes them to conventions and conferences, and she rejoices seeing them grow as professionals.

We spent some time at English Rose Suites, Braemar Hills in Edina, Minnesota. The home was a gem from the outside and a blend of comfort and elegance inside. You may notice a book or a coffee mug not in their proper place, a sign that a happy family lives here. Residents and staff were busy working, playing, and reading; two elders with advanced dementia were absorbed in a serious chat. The ambience bespoke peace, joy, and a hint of lilac fragrance. Jane spends a fortune on essential oils, her aromatic armory always ready to battle any discomfort of body and spirit. Lavender induces dreamless sleep, jasmine calms frayed nerves, and eucalyptus melts away the pains and aches of old age. Each room, in its own way, celebrates the biography of the residents. All through the home, you see a myriad of artifacts, from an antique piano to dainty figurines; they serve as cues that spark memories in a clouded mind, and they reconnect you with a bygone youth filled with dreams, indiscretions, and friendships.

We found camaraderie with one resident, ninety-year-old Mr. Robert Fitzgerald Whitney, decked in vest and tie and looking regal on the crimson settee. His courtly manners matched his aristocratic demeanor—traces from his luxuriant lifestyle of a titan of his day, a master builder who had constructed huge nursing homes. His mind had left him years ago. His family placed him in an affluent, skilled nursing facility where two private nurses kept a vigil twenty-four hours a day. From day one, he seemed restless and got worse by the day. So his family brought him to English Rose Suites. Sitting with us, he waxed eloquent on the history of his family. The CNA Eileen was within earshot and piped in with a crucial detail here and there—an indication of how Jayne makes her staff get to know the resident as a person now, with roots in the past.

We were not finished with Jayne. We asked her, now that she has reached the top, what new directions will she pursue? Branching out? Franchising English Rose Suites? Selling it to eager buyers knocking at the door? Her response aptly summarized the quintessential Jayne

Clairmont. She said, "I have achieved my dream, and I am happy. Branching out into new ventures may stretch me out too far. Bigness is a step towards bureaucracy and impersonality. We have avoided that by cultivating collegiality, informal bonds, and mutual caring. I cannot sell the company to the highest bidder. I did not build this company by myself. The staff and I pooled our strengths, our ideas, and our energies to make ours a success story. Legally, yes, I can sell this business. Morally, I will not, I cannot. I have to think of my residents and my staff. We are a family."

The day we visited her, she was with her accountant, designing her version of employee ownership. Her vision is to give her staff what they have earned by their loyalty and dedication, to motivate them to stay on as partners in compassionate caring of dementia patients.

Employee Stock Option Plans

Employee ownership is a venerable concept, favored by managers and owners with a humanistic bent. It provides living proof that treating workers as humans is good business. Decades of research has established that companies that adopt ESOPs (employee stock option plans) reap measurable benefits. Companies that put ESOPs in place reap a 3 percent faster growth in sales. Their performance measures jump 2 percent per year. ESOP participants have about three times the retirement assets compared to their counterparts and their base pay is 5 to 11 percent higher per year (8.05).

However, research also makes another critical point. Employee ownership is not the magic bullet but one ingredient in the recipe for higher sales, fatter profits, and improved performance. That recipe requires that managers practice what ESOPs promise: employees are owners, and they should be partners in making policy, setting priorities, planning the budget, and sharing information. That is, a heavy-handed management does not let the benefits of ESOPs come to fruition.

Sadly, in long-term care, as of June 2014, only two large nursing home companies were fully employee owned or had ESOPs.

In February 1998, as wished by its founder, the employees of Medicalodges bought the company. Headquartered in Gardner, Kansas, Medicalodges provide skilled care and rehabilitation at twenty-four sites and deploys thousands of workers. The new ESOP trust fund grows in keeping with the company up to the time of retirement. In one telling case, an older, retired CNA needing nursing care became a resident at the home where she had worked; she drew on her ESOP funds to meet the expenses.

Miller's Health Systems operates in Indiana and manages thirty Miller's Merry Manor nursing care centers and nine Miller's assisted living communities. It also leases and operates a hospital transitional unit. The company, founded by Wallace and Connie Miller in 1964, announced in 2006 an ESOP for its three thousand employees. The transition is incomplete, but employees can now share in the company's growth and success by owning a varying percentage of it; the goal is eventually for Miller's Health Systems to be 100 percent employee owned.

Compassion: Heroes and Antiheroes

Think of Jayne Clairmont as a prototype of a humanistic leader. She connects with her staff at the deepest level; she learns what they miss most in life, what they most yearn for. She then creates a workplace culture that teaches them how to care for good people whose minds have left them—a culture that lets them be, become, belong, be their best, and reach beyond.

Now place Jayne, the prototype, on one end of the continuum. On the opposite end, you would place the managers, CFOs, and owners who dehumanized the work and working conditions for Barbara, Dawn, and many other workers. At the two ends of the continuum stand two prototypes of managers who view work and treat workers in a starkly different manner.

On the compassionate end, the person-centered manager sees workers as persons no different from herself or himself. They want to be recognized as persons; they want to be safe, to belong, to be their best, to reach beyond, and to serve. So compassionate managers build an egalitarian culture. They know that exclusion and secrecy are the bulwarks of power, privilege, and hierarchy. So good managers empower, delegate, and share information, strategies, goals, and budgets. They encourage relationships and friendships across roles and departments. They make workers feel wanted and provide them with a sense of ownership, accountability, pride, and loyalty. They create opportunities for workers to do their best, and they celebrate their success. They build teams that cooperate, collaborate, share, serve, help, and teach. They show concern for the workers' personal and family problems.

If hospitals selected managers based on their CAT score (compassion aptitude test score), a test of compassion, we would soon have hospitals where humans and machines would advance far on the road to safety, where one is alert, primed, and ready to prevent risk and to deal wisely with error if it should occur.

On the opposite end of the continuum, you find managers who live by the rules of the market; they see work and worker as economic units; the market determines their value. The free market runs on an amoral logic. Business decisions, by this logic, follow economic principles. Compassion, humanism, morality, and ethics belong to different domains of human life. Their codes should not interfere with the functioning of the free market. In business, you have no friends, only interests.

In truth, work is quintessential human activity with profound significance for every worker—unskilled laborer, professional, manager, or executive. By the sweat of our brow, we earn our daily bread. Work lets us discover our hidden skills, talent, and potential; work is an opportunity to create, to contribute, to grow, to acquire new skills. Work shapes our self-image and identity.

Work reaches its highest ideal when it does not seem like work—when it is rewarding and not burdensome, when your work life and personal life overlap and meld into one happy life. Society accords that privilege to some professions and professionals—professors, judges, artists, for example. In such cases, their personal and professional worlds have no boundaries. Historians and anthropologists have found variants of this holistic ideal across times and cultures.

Industrialization and the market economy introduced a new paradigm of compartmentalized modern life. They redefined work; they separated work from leisure, work from vacation, work from hobby, home from office, weekdays from weekend. This artificial segregation has devalued the lofty meaning of work and has turned it into an odious burden. Thus, come Friday, you hear exclamations of "TGIF" ("Thank God it's Friday") and in the dying hours of the weekend, the familiar lament, "OGIM" ("Oh God, it's Monday").

In an arresting but sad narrative, David Weil, professor, Boston University, shows that it is not technological advances that have degraded work, have killed jobs, and have widened inequality (8.06). Rather, heartless economists have invented a new way of grouping workers as contingent, contract, agency, temp worker. Logically, this classification turns human labor into just another of the marketable goods that you can buy or sell with no thought to the adversity all this may cause to worker and the workers' family.

The nurse in the hospital, the CNA in a nursing home, the FedEx man at the door, the Comcast technician who fixes your cable, the hotel receptionist and room cleaners, and even college adjunct professors—i.e., one in three U.S. workers—are not employed by the companies whose uniform and logo they may wear. They are faceless hirelings herded into a labor pool by intermediaries and given on lease to those companies. These transients pay their own social security, they are often not insured, they seldom collect unemployment compensation, they risk a subminimum wage, wage-theft, or overtime violations, and they work in subpar work conditions and face retaliation at the very reference to a union.

Such dehumanization of the worker is a growing trend both within health care and without.

The Doctor–Patient Democracy

Traditionally, medical paternalism has assigned authority to the doctor and has expected compliance from the patient. Today, patients are involved in medical decision making more than before. In a review of 115 patient participation studies, prior to 2000, only half the studies reported that a majority of patients wished to get involved in medical decision making. But after 2000, 71 percent of studies found a majority of them wished to participate (8.07). Patient participation indicates patient autonomy. The patient needs to understand the options before giving informed consent and making shared decisions. When patients participate, doctors engage in more patient-centered dialogue, and the latter comply more with the agreed-upon regimen.

Many patients, however, avoid participation when they feel they have no real control, when an overbearing doctor does not connect, when the setting is intimidating, or the patient is anxious and disturbed.

Patient empowerment has become a worldwide concern. A report entitled "Patient Power" and published by the Stockholm Network think tank looks at these questions in detail and examines patient associations and their impact on health-care policy in seven key countries. Brazil and Thailand turn out to have the most conducive environments for patient engagement in policy making. (8.08). Denmark has the most empowered patients around Europe.

In 2002, France declared its aim to be a health democracy, in which patient rights and responsibilities include control of their health. Croatia, Hungary, and the Catalan region of Spain have enacted similar regulations. In 2009, British and Australian campaigns were launched to highlight the costs of unhealthy lifestyles and the need for a culture of responsibility (8.09). The European Union has regularly reviewed the question of patients' rights and cooperated with the World Health Organization on this issue since 2005. Collaboration has published a set of standards compiled from participants from fourteen countries around the world, which will help determine the quality of patient decision aids.

On the one hand, managed care has dragged doctors into the marketplace, hemmed them in, and subjected caregiving to market discipline. On the other hand, the rise of consumerism and diffusion of clinical knowledge have encouraged a retail delivery of care services, as is evident in the emergence of new players like Walmart, CVS Caremark, and Walgreens.

Clinical professionals feel besieged; they are frightened away from the path of compassion.

In sum, the workplace profoundly affects the way we define who are. Health-care managers create a workplace that can heal or harm our self-image, support or test your spirit, help or hinder residents and staff to grow and to become.

Part 3. Case Study: Reach Out and Stir Someone

Picture this in your mind.

Elsie is forty-two and has been a home-care aide for over twenty years. Elsie's client Marie is eighty-five. Upon her return home from the hospital, she was unstable and needed to use a wheelchair. One glorious, sunny day, Elsie took Marie out for fresh air. "Pushing the wheelchair several blocks is exactly the exercise I need," Elsie told herself. Then, she pondered, "What about Marie?" So Elsie stopped, helped Marie to get up and stand, holding on to the wheelchair. With neither saying a word, Elsie ceremoniously plopped onto the wheelchair. Marie took deliberate steps to move behind her and, with undue seriousness, piloted her young passenger down the sidewalk. Soon, the incongruity broke through, and they laughed hysterically. Bystanders and passersby made up a friendly audience and, as days passed, became friends with Elsie and Marie. By week's end, things changed: Marie went from wheelchair to walker, her bond with Elsie cemented, and they made new friends in the neighborhood.

You may wonder what a nursing home state surveyor may have to say about this happenstance. However, you do not have to doubt how Ms. Karen Love would react—Karen mentored Elsie in the therapeutic engagement technique, which she authored.

Street smarts and a spoonful of sugar

Karen Love, an expert in assisted living, has a mind that runs on its own track. She does not seek new answers to old questions; rather, she rephrases the questions. When *The Kiplinger Letter* learned that Karen had brought a recalcitrant auto shop to its knees but then had turned its manager into her "new best friend," the editor put Karen on its cover page and titled the story, "Have a Complaint? Street Smarts and a Spoonful of Sugar Can Get Results."

Karen had worked in the assisted living field as both staff and manager. She saw its hidden flaws close-up; when her career path changed, she founded CCAL, a quality-advocacy coalition in assisted living. She enrolled her kids in a Montessori preschool and watched the tykes grow into little Einsteins; their study and play merged, and they seemed as eager for school as to stay home. These Montessori outcomes planted an idea: "If Montessori has that effect on kids," her thought whispered, "why don't you try it on the elders?" That thought matured and gave birth to therapeutic engagement. Karen used the Montessori approach to children's education to design therapeutic engagement as a way to release the caged spirit within people with dementia.

The Montessori method is named after an Italian physician and educator, Maria Montessori (1870–1952). Based on her work with children, she argued that the child's true normal nature needs freedom to blossom; it needs a teacher who creates a conducive environment, uses proper learning tools, guides self-directed learning, and directs peer-shared activity. A mountain of research has proven her right. Of the seven thousand Montessori schools worldwide, over half are in the United States.

Karen borrowed from Montessori's key insights to design therapeutic engagement. In Montessori, you assume that a person lies hidden within a child, waiting to grow, perhaps, into a Nobel Prize winner. The role of a Montessori teacher is to clear the clutter that blocks that growth, to coax that genius to emerge through self-discovery in an appropriate climate.

The Treasure Hidden in a Shell

In therapeutic engagement, Karen assumes the opposite. The elderly woman you meet, Karen tells you, is more than what your eyes behold, she is actually the sum total of all her past and present; she carries within her all her past struggles, triumphs, joys, and tears.

A dependent, confused nursing home resident, now a mere shell of her earlier triumphant self, houses inside that shell a unique biography, fond experiences, treasured mementos, and rich memories. Montessori detects in every child a yearning for room to grow and to achieve; therapeutic engagement detects in every dependent elder a yearning for recognition of what one has been, has achieved, and has contributed. Karen taught Elsie to reach out behind the aging shell, to touch something meaningful in her client's rich life and biography, and to draw the elder into a therapeutic engagement.

This conviction led Karen to Walmart; she pushed her shopping cart down the aisles and collected the teaching aids she would use in training caregivers—skeins of knitting wool, glass beads, wigs, decks of cards, and other things. She found that the color, feel, shape, and smells of these low-tech teaching aids stirred something inside a confused elder—they evoked memories and brought to life their long-forgotten experiences.

Karen has used her approach in nursing homes, adult day care centers, and in-home care to train staff and family caregivers. The resulting physical, mental, and social therapeutic benefits have been video-recorded and testified to by families, staff, and research results of studies supported, among others, by the Virginia Alzheimer's and Related Diseases Research Fund, the National Institute on Aging, and the Agency on Aging.

Although you find Karen talking policy with policy makers and partnering in research with academics, she is truly herself—warm, friendly, and caring—in the company of caregivers giving care. Wherever she might be in person, her imagination roams the universe, searching for low-tech devices to help people with dementia live fuller lives. She is so successful at it that the National Institute on Aging funded her latest product, Fit Kits, a unique collection of items designed to stimulate and engage a person with dementia at any stage.

CHAPTER 9

The Human Need and Right to Belong

To Relate, to Connect, to Love, to Be Wanted

Piglet sidled up to Pooh from behind. "Pooh?" he whispered.
"Yes, Piglet?"
"Nothing," said Piglet, taking Pooh's hand.
"I just wanted to be sure of you."
—*A. A. Milne*

Humans gaze at the sky and contemplate the stars out of nostalgia. We are connected to the heavens. The ocean bed, the mountaintops, and the open sky have shaped our bodies and minds over three million years.

Our lust for life, our yearning to be our own self, to be master of our destiny, to be our best, to transcend, and to belong—these are primal forces, still raw and not fully tamed. Our drives and passions have yet to be fully domesticated. "We are all genetic chimeras," E. O. Wilson, Harvard sociobiology professor emeritus, has written. "We are at once saints and sinners, champions of the truth and hypocrites—because of the way our species originated across millions of years of biological evolution."

Our evolutionary contradictions play out most prominently in the health-care arena. Health care is highly sophisticated, but it fails to ensure our safety. Our managers are schooled to lead and mentor, but they heed the market and compromise the humanity of the caregiver. We are wired to belong, to relate, and to love, but rampant distrust, malpractice threat, and defensive medicine dog us the day long.

This chapter addresses some of these contradictions in health care. We point out the trials and tribulations they create.

Humans are hardwired to connect with the world, to relate to people, and to belong to groups. Initially, our loyalty was to ourselves and to our immediate family. Through history, we have broadened the circle of those we love. Nature has ordained that as our social affiliation broadens and deepens, we improve in health, body, mind, and soul. Affiliation by marriage, religion, ethnicity leads to a longer life and a deeper life satisfaction.

Part 1. Human Solidarity and Human Well-Being

The craving for companionship is so natural and so deeply ingrained that human connections are indispensable for our health and well-being. The extreme opposite of social interaction is social isolation. Society has used solitary confinement to punish deviant behavior; terrorists have used it as an effective tool of torture.

Émile Durkheim launched sociology as a science with his landmark study of social integration. He wanted to know how a person's bond to one's group affected suicide. In 1869, he mapped out the suicide rate in France (135 per million), England (67 per million), and Denmark (277 per million) (9.01).

Durkheim's map revealed the following:

- Suicide rates are higher in men than in women, higher among singles than among married, and higher for those without children than those with children.
- Suicide rates are higher among Protestants than Catholics and Jews.
- Suicide rates are higher among civilians than soldiers and higher in times of peace than in times of war.
- Suicide rates are higher in Scandinavian countries.
- Suicide rates are higher among the more educated.

Durkheim concluded that suicide may be an individual act, but the social context directly affects it. In the 1970s, researchers pursued that theme with vigor—how social connectedness affects human health. Such investigations mushroomed in the 1980s. To date, research has firmly established that social links are powerful predictors of human and animal health, mortality, and longevity. Positive social engagement encourages healthy behavior. Social relationships themselves independently influence health and mortality.

Social Solidarity and Healthy Habits

In 1965, Berkman and Breslow initiated a pioneering prospective study of a sample of 6,928 people in Alameda County, California (9.02). The study focused on seven health habits that predict health and mortality: (1) never smoked, (2) less than five alcoholic drinks at one sitting, (3) sleeping seven to eight hours a night, (4) exercising, (5) maintaining desirable weight for height, (6) avoiding snacks between meals, and (7) eating breakfast regularly. The Alameda 7 study has continued and has been duplicated and expanded upon. Over the years, these studies have reached firm conclusions (9.03).

Although two of the seven, namely, snacking between meals and eating breakfast regularly, have not shown to influence health in all studies, the five others have proven to be powerful determinants of health. Those practicing zero to three of the seven health habits live to sixty-seven years. Those following four to five practices live to seventy-three, and those following six to seven practices live to seventy-eight. Adults with coronary artery disease die of cardiac death 2.4 times more often when they are socially isolated than when they are socially connected.

Social solidarity—especially marital and religious solidarity—promotes the adoption of the seven health-related practices; they independently boost physical and mental well-being (9.04).

Married people are less ill and disabled; their survival rate is greater for some illnesses (9.05). Nine out of ten married women alive at age forty-eight will be alive at age sixty-five; by contrast, eight out of ten never-married women would survive to age sixty-five. A more pronounced difference shows up among men: nine out of ten married men versus only six out of ten never married at the age of forty-eight will reach age sixty-five (9.06). Marital life lowers the risk of cardiovascular disease, chronic conditions, mobility limitations, low self-rated health, and depressive symptoms (9.07).

Being married and staying married to the same person make for better mental health. After marriage, emotional well-being increases; it declines following the end of a union (9.08). Through the decades, researchers have documented that married men are happier than men who have never married or are divorced (9.09). Married people enjoy the highest emotional and physical satisfaction with sex. Noncohabiting singles have the least satisfaction, and cohabiters fall somewhere in between (9.10).

Religion improves health and longevity. It knits people into a community and leads to the adoption of the seven health practices. Religious involvement lowers the risk of heart disease, stroke, hypertension, cancer, and gastrointestinal disease. Members of stricter religious denominations reap higher benefits (9.11). At the age of twenty, church attendees can look forward to a life seven years longer than those who never attend church. Religious activity brings families together in closer and deeper ties (9.12). The nonreligious are less satisfied with sex than are frequent churchgoers (9.13). Couples who pray together experience more ecstasy in their sex lives (9.14).

Domestic violence prevails more among cohabitors than among the married (9.15). About 14 percent of cohabitors say that they or their mate hit, shoved, or threw things at their partner during the past year, compared to 5 percent of those who are formally married. The difference declines when age, education, and race are held constant. Violence occurs less between engaged cohabiting couples than between uncommitted cohabitors (9.16).

The Social Brain

"We are all curious collages, weird little planetoids that grow by accreting other people's habits and ideas and styles and tics and jokes and phrases and tunes and hopes and fears as if they were meteorites that came soaring out of the blue, collided with us, and stuck.

"The brain is exquisitely social, and emotions are its fundamental language. Through them we become integrated and develop an emergent resonance with the internal state of the other. When we work with relationship, we work with brain structure. Relationship stimulates us and is essential in our development."

—Douglas Hofstadter, 2011

Blessed Are the Married and the God-Fearing

Why do marriage and religion contribute to our well-being? Social connections keep one healthy for obvious reasons. First, intimacy and friendship create a body chemistry that supports a healthy body and mind; health of body and mind, in turn, lead to happiness, satisfaction, and physical delight. Second, a loving bond evokes a mutual urge to support, aid, and empathize. A caring partner is your virtual guardian angel, alert and concerned about your welfare, urging you to keep to the road of moderation and a healthy lifestyle.

Third, marital solidarity instills accountability and obligations to your dear ones. You owe it to your family to take care of yourself and to avoid risky behavior, situations, and people. Fourth, married life demands discipline, accommodation, and a routine that bridles the unregulated practices of premarital days. The discipline of marital life tames your wild streak and sets you on route Alamedas 7, with the promise of a healthier, longer life. Fifth, marriage enriches your social network and connects you to new people—like your in-laws.

Like marriage, religion is an integrative force. Religious groups create occasions for people to meet, to socialize, to make friends, to lend a helping hand. Some religions limit the use of alcohol, tobacco, caffeine, and other harmful foods. Frequent church attendees boast larger social networks and relationships that are more meaningful. Religious belief, ritual, and services are welcome comfort in times of pain, defeat, bereavement, and illness (9.17). Religious traditions help socialize children into healthy behaviors. They add meaning and purpose in old age (9.18).

There is a dark side, however. Both married and religious life risk harm to humans, especially when the commitment is soft (9.19). Spouse abuse and family conflict trigger adverse immunological changes, increasing the risk of illness. So too, far too often, the good functions of religion turn into harmful dysfunctions. Religious solidarity has bred fanaticism, and more blood has been shed in the name of religion than in any other. Religious beliefs and codes have nurtured the guilt complex, anxiety, and infantilism. Religion has too often degraded women and has kept them trapped them into exploitative marital bondage.

Caring for dear ones may also involve personal health costs. Caring for an impaired spouse imposes strains and increases physical and mental distress (9.20). Caregiver stress affects interactions with the care receiver (9.21).

Social and economic factors determine forty percent of human health (9.22). Overwhelming evidence leaves no doubt that social connectedness profoundly affects human health and well-being. Friends, family, marriage and religion encourage health-promoting behaviors and add to longevity.

Part 2. Compassion in Health Care

Of all the forms that humans take, by far the most glorious is compassion. Compassion lies at the heart of medicine; it elevates the practice of medicine to an art, and it sublimates the doctor-patient encounter into a sacred bond.

James R. Doty, MD, is a professor of neurosurgery at Stanford University and the founder and director of the Center for Compassion and Altruism Research and Education. He spoke of a heartwarming encounter between Tibetan monks and scientists studying the link between meditation and compassion (9.23). The researchers were placing the electroencephalography electrode cap on a monk's head. The monks laughed, but not because the cap looked funny. A monk explained, "Everyone knows that compassion isn't in the head. It's in the heart."

Dr. Doty, the leader in the science of compassion, said, "Indeed, it is through the heart that we are connected with others… Scientists around the world have now demonstrated that, in great part, the monk was correct." Sudden cardiac death is caused by due decreased vagal tone that throws the heart rate out of gear; releases more cortisol, the stress hormone; and decreases immune function.

He explains, the vagus nerve arises in the brain stem and innervates many organs, especially the heart. Compassionate action tones up the vagus nerve, which lowers stress. It calms you, lowers your heart rate, and inclines you to feel empathy. Just two of compassion practice can lower biological symptoms of stress and improve the biological markers of immune function.

Dr. Doty has found that compassion dramatically activates the brain areas associated with food and sex. Receiving money and giving money to charity activate these. When looking for mates, men may value physical attractiveness and women may value a stable provider, but far beyond any other trait, both sexes value kindness and compassion in a partner. Girls release oxytocin (the cuddle or love hormone related to bonding behavior) significantly more when speaking to their mother in person or over the phone rather than when texting her. Ever-increasing data show that when we care for others and feel close to them, we improve our own health and even our longevity. We are designed to care and to connect. By helping others, we help ourselves.

Compassion seems to possess magical powers. Compassion moves us to the depth when we experience it, when we practice it, or even when we merely witness it. It transmutes the link between caregiver and care receiver, imbues it with meaning, and gives it a power to transform suffering and to hasten healing. Its transcendent nature makes compassionate giving satisfying in itself. Compassion is its own reward. Studies show that for caregivers in every sector and at every level, relationships are of paramount value, and a compassionate workplace is the ultimate prize.

A study of 685 nursing home administrators (NHAs) around the nation drew attention to the importance of human connections as nursing home managers (9.24). A hefty 64 percent of NHAs were satisfied with their role, and 13 percent were highly satisfied. Their relations with residents, families, and staff were the most important sources of their satisfaction.

One NHA commented, "My greatest reward is I make a difference in people's lives, to hear families say that we care." Another commented, "It is 7:00 p.m. and I have dealt with paperwork, visited with a few of my residents and families, talked to some staff, and I am still not done. I love the business of caring for others and it is why I have stayed so many years."

Relationships are very important for a nurse-leader. In her work, the bonds she helps create with and among residents, staff members, families, and colleagues are a measure of her success. A survey of nursing home directors of nursing (DONs) revealed that DONs experience a high level of satisfaction with their work (9.25). Their satisfaction borders on exuberance: 84 percent agreed or strongly agreed that they are overall satisfied. Being a nurse-leader is a rewarding experience for a great number of DONs. Relationships were a fount of strength and support and satisfaction. Relationships showed up in the top seven out of the seventeen important sources of a DON's satisfaction. Inadequate salary, insufficient professional growth, a lack of tools to manage—these problems frustrate a DON, but not as much as the absence of warm relations in the workplace.

Compassion and caregiving are integral to a DON's calling. What satisfies her most is resident care (52 percent) and knowing that she makes a difference in people's lives (47 percent). "My greatest reward," said one DON, "is to know the difference I make in people's lives, in seeing the progress residents make, and watching staff develop professionally. Nothing is more gratifying than the feeble 'Thank you, honey,' the touch of a frail hand, or the heartwarming smiles I am blessed with every day."

Compassion assumes great significance in long-term care management. It is an indispensable element in the commitment of the caregiving staff. MIV/National Research has archives of satisfaction data on millions of CNAs in thousands of nursing homes in the USA. Researchers who have mine that data, report that, year after year, and regardless of the type, size and location of their nursing home, CNAs say they get their highest satisfaction from the simple fact that their job lets them make a difference in the lives of residents. Altruism is a shining trait of a nursing home CNA.

As in long-term care, compassion and relational ties are the pathway to healing, well-being, and satisfaction in acute care. The Hippocratic Oath says simply, "I will remember that… warmth, sympathy, and understanding may outweigh the surgeon's knife or the chemist's drug."

Bernard Lown, MD, one of the greatest cardiologists, inventor of the defibrillator, and a Nobel laureate, authored a classic, *The Lost Arts of Healing: Practicing Compassion in Medicine* (9.26). He points to tiny gestures that have a mighty impact. Even just attentive listening conveys compassion and creates a healing relationship; it yields better diagnosis, better adherence to regimen, and faster recovery at levels of neurology, immunology, and endocrinology. He advocates a culture of compassionate care. In such a culture, insensitivity and rudeness are anathema; people's manners, etiquette, dress, and speech reflect and affirm the genuine feelings of respect, hospitality, and attentiveness.

Danielle Ofri, in her book *What Doctors Feel: How Emotions Affect the Practice of Medicine* (9.27), refers with admiration to her mentors of a bygone era. They were white men-doctors in starched shirts and bow ties that were schooled in lily-white settings in an age before *diversity* became politically correct. Yet they were culturally aware, their old-fashioned doctoring made them approach the bedside as a sacred act. "They examined each patient—whether a homeless Ecuadorian alcoholic or a veiled Muslim woman or a visiting Swiss diplomat—with a thoroughness that in itself exuded respect."

She speaks of Dr. Spenser, of his blustering style and of a heart soaked in compassion. He mentored the young medics-to-be on compassion. He would drag a metal stool to the exam table, swivel it down to the lowest level and would sit on it with his head level to the exam table. Then he would say, "Whenever you speak to a patient, you seat yourself at the patient's level or lower. You never hover over them high and mighty. They are the ones who are sick. They run the interview, not you."

Illness intensifies the need for human connection, especially in a cold and sterile hospital setting. For the helpless patient, a compassionate caregiver is a godsend—whose reassuring presence, soothing touch, and caring hasten recovery and healing more surely than the cold potency of the formulary.

In general, compassion helps prevent illness and facilitates disease management as well as self-care skills (9.28). Compassion makes a patient feel secure, lowers cortisol levels, and speeds wound healing. Emotionally disturbed patients heal slower. Researchers created tiny uniform blisters on the arms of forty-two married couples. In couples with high levels of hostility, healing slowed to 60 percent and took two days more than for couples with low hostility. That gap also showed up in their biochemistry (cytokine). A review of twenty-one studies concluded that a satisfying doctor-patient interaction increases physical functions and emotional health and decreases pain. Myocardial infarction patients who experience compassion in the hospital have better health and significantly lower mortality rate in the first year after discharge (9.29).

The retreat of compassion deals the cruelest blow to the doctor-patient bond that has been regarded inviolable from ages past. The Schwartz Center for Compassionate Healthcare reports on the survey of 800 recently hospitalized patients and 510 physicians. Both groups agreed that compassionate care is very important to successful medical treatment. However, only 53 percent of patients and 58 percent of physicians said that the health-care system generally provides compassionate care. When asked about compassionate care at the individual level, 78 percent of physicians said that most health-care professionals provide compassionate care, but only 54 percent of patients said that they do.

A typical physician experiences about 150,000 patient encounters in her or his career. Fifty-three (53) percent of doctors say they spend less time with their patients than they want to. Fifty-five (55) percent complain the system does not allow them to provide emotional support. Actually, visits with internists, family doctors, and pediatricians increased by about two and a half minutes. The average physician visit in 2010 across specialties lasted 20.8 minutes with the patient compared to 16.3 minutes in 1991–1992 and 18.9 minutes in 2000. "When I was a house surgeon, the average length-of-stay… was eight to nine days. Now it is three-and-a-half. Then we had the luxury of waiting three or four days for trust to build".

Longer visits still frustrate patients when doctors do not listen and when they interrupt. In one 1999 study, one in four patients got to finish their statement; doctors let patients speak for only twenty-three seconds before breaking in (9.30). In a 2001 study, patients were interrupted after twelve seconds by the doctor, a beeper, or a knock on the door (9.31).

The distance between doctor and patient deprives the doctor of firsthand knowledge of the patient. Too often, it is not the clinician but a subordinate who takes the patient's history. Almost one in three hospital patients do not know the lead doctor in charge of their care.

In 1996, only half of hospitalized Medicare patients received care from a clinician who had seen them in the previous year. In 2006, that percentage had dropped to 40 percent (9.32). Close to two in three hospitalized patients are not in touch with their usual doctor while they are in the hospital. One in three adults do not inform their doctor that they underuse medication for chronic conditions (9.33). At discharge from hospital, less than half of patients know their diagnosis or their medications.

Short visits, little dialogue, and no regular ongoing communication frustrate both patients and doctors, but neither feel they can control a system with a mind of its own. Even primary care doctors (especially those in group practice) bend to the demands of managed care.

Money is part of the calculus. Students enter medical school with high ideals and finish twelve years later with an average of $166,750 of medical school debt to be paid over thirty years at 7.5 percent interest for a total cost of $419,738. And these numbers are from 2012, a year when more than one in four doctors saw a cut in pay. So to avoid an income drop, doctors attend to four patients an hour instead of three (9.34).

On every measure, it seems that doctor and patient have drifted apart. Their meetings have become ritual, they don't lead to inter-personal knowledge, concern or bonds.

Patients feel cheated when they are put on the waiting list, when they barely get enough time with the doctor, and don't get a chance to say what they have to say. As a patient, you say to yourself that you waited three months to get this appointment—you took time off work for it. And all you get is three minutes? The doctor is driven by the assigned quota: "I have only ten minutes. I better get all the patient info I need."

One is on Mars, the other on Venus; they communicate on different wavelengths.

From Trust to Antipathy

The personal doctor–patient encounter is unique in that it is tinged with primal emotions, and it carries a sacred aura—just the right mix for trust to turn into antipathy. The ugliest perversion of compassion is malpractice litigation.

One out of two neurosurgeons and one in three orthopedic surgeons, emergency physicians, and trauma surgeons are sued each year. Eighty-one (81) percent of medical residents see every patient as a potential lawsuit. Ninety-three (93) percent of physicians admit practicing some form of defensive medicine, costing about $200 billion a year. (9.35).

Research spanning from 1995 to 2005 shows that ineffective team communication is the root cause for nearly 66 percent of all medical errors for that period (9.36). Add to that the physical and emotional gulf that has grown between the doctor and patient, which results in a fertile ground for malpractice. As early as 1973, poor physician-patient relationship were known to cause 71 percent of the malpractice claims. Patients who sue fit a profile: they have sued before; their visits with the doctor lasted less than ten minutes; they felt rushed or ignored, not listened to, and not given adequate explanations for tests; their satisfaction was not high; and they saw the doctor as unconcerned, inaccessible, and not eager to communicate (9.37). Increasingly, doctors view patients as potential adversaries. In one study, three-fourths of the specialists had such a view. One in three litigations refer to inattentiveness, discourtesy and rudeness, a general breakdown in communication, and inadequate information (9.38).

Abraham Verghese observes, "Patients who like their doctors don't sue, no matter what their lawyer says... Patients sue when their feelings are ignored or when they are angered by lack of genuine concern for their welfare… A sound physician-patient relationship is a powerful antidote to frivolous lawsuits" (9.39).

To conclude, the irony stands out stark and clear: at a time when the world takes giant steps in advancing communication and networking technology, communication breakdown stalks health care and results in widespread medical errors and injuries. Strained relationships have leeched out the humane element in therapeutic encounters, have turned trust to antipathy, and have frustrated the fundamental right of care receivers and caregivers to belong, to connect, and to love.

Models and Exemplars: The Many Faces of Compassion

James Fowler at the University of California, San Diego, found that a single act of kindness typically inspired several more acts of generosity (9.40). As a recipient of a kind act, you tend to act kindly toward others, and those recipients act kindly in turn, in a chain reaction academics label as *upstream reciprocity*. Kindness also radiates laterally. A witness to an altruistic act is moved to act generously to others. When Harvard students watched a film about Mother Theresa, the number of protective antibodies in their saliva surged; when the students were asked to focus on times when they'd been loved by or shown love to others, their antibody levels stayed elevated for an hour (9.41).

Christian Smith and Hilary Davidson write about *The Paradox of Generosity: Giving We Receive, Grasping We Lose*. Small acts of kindness can have an oversize impact: dropping a quarter into an expired parking meter, paying for a cup of coffee and reserving it for a homeless person, paying off a stranger's layaway balance at Walmart, or persuading your child to donate to homeless children half of what the child would receive as Christmas presents.

The need for kindness and empathy takes on a deep significance in times of illness (9.42). Steve Schalchlin, accomplished musician, songwriter, and AIDS activist, was the 2000 Jonathan J. King lecturer at a Stanford University teach-in. He walked to the front of hundreds of physicians and caregivers and began singing about facing death at a young age: "Living in the Bonus Round."

"If you're expecting facts and figures, you won't find any," Schalchlin told his audience. Instead, he thanked them "for being physicians, for caring… thank you for taking five extra seconds to tell a patient they look really good today." He recalled, late one night, four years ago, as he lay desperately ill and his will to live was at its lowest, a young nurse came into his hospital room. She sat with him, took his hand, and quietly said, "You know, you're our favorite patient on this floor." That kind, compassionate act, Mr. Schalchlin told them, rekindled his spirit and sparked his will to live.

Our research and fieldwork rewarded us with unanticipated encounters with compassion. The following is a small sample (9.43).

- At a Planetree hospital, Lori, a nurse, came in for a job interview at 7:30 a.m., a bit ahead of time. In the lobby, she looked around to get oriented when a kindly gentleman walked up and greeted her warmly. "Good morning! May I help you?" Before he walked with her to her interview in the New Friends Room 3, he offered her freshly brewed coffee. It was not until the end of her interview that Lori learned that the gentleman who welcomed her and offered her coffee was the hospital CEO!

- "We walked into our daughter's hospital room and found the chief resident sitting beside her crib, reading her *Harold and the Purple Crayon*, one of her favorite books. No other doctor had given this attention to her as a person, a child, a human being who had just been diagnosed with stage 4 neuroblastoma."

- "We had been home three days after an out-of-state visit with a specialist who diagnosed our son's rare medical condition. The doctor called. He said he had done nothing for those three days but think about my son and researched his disorder. He had discovered some possible treatments. He would call our son's doctors and share his findings. He did, and he has continued to work with our pediatrician, neurologist, cardiologist, pulmonologist, and orthopedist over the last two years. Nothing could have prepared us for the outstanding collaborative relationship we have developed."

- "We first met Sister C the day of our son's first major surgery. She appeared at his bedside before 6:00 a.m. to pray with us before he was brought to pre-op. Since that day, she has found us either in person or by note every time we have been back in the hospital. I've never had to ask for her. I recall sitting in the medical surgical ICU one day, exhausted from the previous day's events. I looked up, and there she was."

- "Our daughter's geneticist had some test results to share with us. He told us she had Prader-Willi syndrome. He told us that because of this rare, complex syndrome, she would never go to college, have children of her own, or live independently. All my dreams for my only child were destroyed in this twenty-minute office visit. That's not all I remember. I remember this famous physician coming out from behind his desk and sitting next to us. I remember him telling us not only what was going to go wrong with our dreams for our daughter but also what we could expect to go right, that someday she would walk, talk, relate to us, and achieve things we didn't think possible. 'The one guarantee I can make,' he said, 'is that she's going to surprise you. '

"What I remember most is that at one point, he laid his hand on my arm to comfort me. And it did. That human gesture confirmed for me that he was not only brilliant but wise. I know, because we've talked about it since, that he considered giving me that comfort as important a part of taking care of my daughter as giving a correct diagnosis."

- Cameo, the new life enrichment coordinator at a nursing home, was curious; Brenda, a restorative aide, would arrive early before her shift each day and would go to the room of Mrs. McDermott. Mrs. M was contracted, frail, and near the end of her fight with Alzheimer's disease. She was unable to take part in the restorative exercises led by the aide. Cameo watched Brenda walk into the room with a curling iron, comb, and hairspray. She gently combed, curled, and styled Mrs. M's hair. Brenda had learned from Mrs. M's daughter that her mother had always taken great care of her appearance. As Brenda worked on her hair, Mrs. M's pleasure was evident. She gently turned toward Brenda and smiled; her breathing slowed, and she drifted into a deep, snoring sleep. That was Cameo's second week working in long-term care. Brenda's simple but powerful act of kindness toward one who could not even say "Thank you" both humbled and enriched Cameo.

CHAPTER 10

The Human Need and Right to Be Your Best

When There Is No Way Out, There Is Always a Way Through

Leonardo's Mona Lisa is just a thousand thousand smears of paint. Michelangelo's David is just a million hits with a hammer. We're all of us a million bits put together the right way.
—*Chuck Palahniuk*

Man is not destroyed by suffering; he is destroyed by suffering without meaning.
—*Viktor Frankl*

"It was 5:15 a.m. as I looked out on Lake Michigan. It was like glass. I took my kayak about a mile out on the gentle smoothness of the lake, far from any sound," said Victor Strecher, a professor at the University of Michigan (10.01). He had spent several months here amid the expanse of water and nature's beauty. He was looking for solace and comfort as he grieved the terrible loss in 2010 of Julia, his nineteen-year-old daughter, stricken as a baby by a virus that damaged her heart and a recipient of two heart transplants. This morning, he was up early after a profound dream in which Julia had visited him.

Out on the lake as the sun rose over the horizon and turned the water to gold, he relived his dream. "I felt Julia in me, telling my heart that I needed to 'get over it.'"

The tragedy had crippled him. His success as an academic, a researcher, and winner of honors and awards could not pull him away from the grip of profound sadness.

Now Julia was telling him to "get over it," to "get over my ego—and to find a new, transcending purpose in my life… The tenuous nature of Julia's life reminded me of the finite years in my own life and that became my change agent."

Now, Strecher is reengaged with life; he promotes health via the Internet and has written about the transforming power of meaning and purpose in life in his book *On Purpose*. He founded the Center for Health Communications Research and Health Media. Victor Strecher lives a full life. He quotes Simone De Beauvoir: "There is only one solution if old age is not to become an absurd parody of our former life, and that is to go on pursuing ends that give our existence a meaning."

He asked, "Can you say, 'I'm so happy I could die now?' Julia could. I can. Especially today. This was Julia's gift to me."

Strecher's story points to two central themes in the humanistic view of life that we discuss in this chapter. First, a dividing line runs through the life most of us lead; in truth, it is a gap between the life we actually live and the more rewarding life we are called to live. Oscar Wilde said it pithily, "To live is the rarest thing in the world. Most people exist, that is all."

Second, the mental distress and depression that afflict moderns stem mostly from the empty life they lead, i.e., a life without direction, without meaning, or without purpose. As Viktor Frankl phrased it, "Those who have a 'why' to live, can bear with almost any 'how'." Following up on these themes, we point to the heights caregivers soar when let to spread their wings.

This chapter examines the human craving for self-fulfillment and a meaningful life. We refer to direct caregivers in long-term care to drive home the point that contrary to the public prejudice, materialistic motivation is not what drives behavior of the lower income groups. Rather, evidence shows that low-status workers yearn to achieve and to have a purpose in life, at least as much as those in the executive ranks do. We illustrate how good managers empower the workers to be their best. Finally, we address the irony of the end of life. We vigorously strive to live a fulfilling and purposeful life, while out of sight, the prevalent culture of death makes it likely that most of us will die a meaningless death, in a way we do not wish or want.

Part 1. Self-Actualization and Health Care

Psychology refers to our primal urge to grow as self-actualization, a label introduced by the gestalt psychologist Kurt Goldstein (1878–1965) in his 1939 book *The Organism*. Carl Rogers (1902–1987) embraced it in his client-centered therapy. Carl Jung (1875–1961) developed aspects of it in his notion of individuation.

A discussion about self-actualization inevitably invokes Abraham Maslow (1908–1970). Maslow challenged the behaviorist image of humans as conditioned lab rats. He opposed the empiricist reduction of human life to quantifiable activity. He noted that Freud had supplied the sick half of psychology; he would fill out the healthy half (10.02). Then, in 1946, logotherapy of Viktor Frankl (1905–1997) gave a strong boost to positive psychology.

Positive psychology views our yearning to become everything we are capable of becoming as distinctive to human life. In self-actualization, a person takes full advantage of her or his talents. In order to compile the characteristics of a self-actualized person, Maslow studied a sample from the admired, great self-actualized persons in history and in his times. The sample included Thomas Jefferson, Abraham Lincoln, Albert Einstein, William James, Aldous Huxley, Gandhi, Beethoven, and Eleanor Roosevelt. Thus, he describes self-actualization as the peak of human performance, as human beings at their very best. Self-actualization displays these traits.

In general, a self-actualized person

- accepts oneself and others as they are;
- maintains deep and meaningful relationships;
- demonstrates empathy and compassion for others;
- has a strong sense of personal ethics and responsibility;
- is thoughtful, philosophical, and has a sense of humor;
- is realistic, logical, and rational;
- is autonomous and independent;
- is open, unconventional, and spontaneous;
- values privacy and enjoys solitude;
- leads a purposeful life and enjoys the journey; and
- enjoys frequent peak experiences—moments of profound happiness.

Notice how comprehensive in scope these traits are. They overlap and span across the five human needs. Self-actualization in its fullness is a lofty level of existence, rarely achieved by many, perhaps by only 1 percent of adults, who, according to Maslow, may not remain in that state all the time. Not all people seek self-actualization. Many merely exist; they do not live.

Reservoir of Possibilities

Long-term care institutions are a wasteland of skills and talent. Too many advocates of nursing-home residents act as if old age dries up the human need to grow and achieve. The residents in a nursing home were, in younger days, mothers, fathers, teachers, mentors, counselors, and guides. They took pride in childrearing, in setting an elegant dinner table, baking the best chocolate chip cookies in the neighborhood, and lending a helping hand or ear to their neighbor.

A nursing home is a reservoir of wisdom, experience, well-honed skills, and talent. Despite its stated goal of person-centered care, many a nursing home fails to create the context for residents to express their talent, to showcase their skills, to teach the next generation. In nursing homes in Holland, we witnessed staff wheeling into the kitchen area women residents with coiffed hairdos and pearls. They sat around the table, cheerfully peeling potatoes or shelling beans or dicing carrots for their evening dinner. It was quite a chatty group swapping stories, gossip, and culinary tips.

Such commonsensical practices like letting residents help in the kitchen or setting the table are unthinkable in the United States because regulations forbid them, because of fear of infection, because a for-profit nursing home avoids any appearance of exploitation of vulnerable seniors, and because as ever, the sword of liability hangs over your head. Thus, the exceptions to this trend stand out as stellar exemplars.

- Joey was apathetic, lethargic, and uninterested in activity programs in the rehab center. When the activity director learned that in his youth in Italy, Joey restored artwork inside cathedrals, she brought him a touch screen tablet and a blunt-tip paintbrush with a lengthened handle. She installed on the tablet a painting program and turned on Italian music.

Joey immediately came alive. The paintbrush rediscovered his identity—Joey flourished the paintbrush as a pro. He began to paint in strategic, short, well-thought-out strokes. His face was utter concentration and focus. In sonorous soprano, he sang along with the music in the background. Joey seemed not to tire. He sang, he painted, and he took short breaks but was always back, wielding the paintbrush and belting out Italian operas.

- Delphina, an alert CNA, heard Lilly, the resident she cared for, reminisce about her days on the stage. Delphina spoke to her DON. And that initiated a remarkable program. The staff and residents formed an actor's club. They chose a play, selected the cast, and kept practicing every Tuesday. The elders would read their script rather than recite it by heart. They staged the play for the community around the nursing home. The event was such a success the residents repeated that feat twice a year for the appreciative audience. Well-known documentaries like Young@Heart Chorus have recorded variations on the same theme (10.03).

- A nursing home in Virginia helped Alice, a resident and a former juvenile court judge, to continue her professional role. Her regal looks, sophisticated demeanor, and Solomonic approach elevated her to the status of the judge in the nursing home. Managers, staff, and residents brought to her disputes, suspicions, and disagreements and abided by her thoughtful and balanced pronouncements.

- CNA Kathy thought to herself, "I love working with grandmas. They tell me the joy they experienced seeing their grandkids grow into beautiful young people. How much they miss the laughter and play of little kids! And my little toddler has never had a grandma or a grandpa."

- Now, Kathy's son, Jimmy, accompanies her often to the nursing home. He has many grandparents now—so many that that he cannot count them. He enjoys the way they fuss over him. They wait for him to come. They are always ready to play with him and happy when he brings them cookies. This cross-generational camaraderie adds meaning to the lives of the elders and fun to the toddler's life.

- Nurse Anita found a way to awaken the spirit within a withdrawn and depressed resident, Cecilia. A little probing revealed that Cecilia was accomplished at crocheting. The next day, Anita went to work with yellow yarn and needles. At day's end, when the bustle had given way to a peaceful evening, Anita sat by Cecilia's side. Pleadingly she asked Cecilia if she would be her teacher and give her lessons in crocheting. Of course, Cecilia rose to the occasion. It took weeks, but the teacher gradually emerged out of her shell and began to attend group events. Whatever happened to the things they crocheted? That nice detail is missing in this story.

Caregivers Spread Their Wings

Two CNAs, Rose and Annette, were seated at a plush desk across from state representative JW. Inside the state Capitol, Olympia, Washington, the air was warm after the day's heated debate in the House of Representatives. The face-off was on the proposed shift of budgetary funds from nursing homes to the salmon fish industry. Annette and Rose were there, making a case for the nursing homes.

JW, the legislator, convincingly listed the reasons for the two constituents seated across his desk as to why he favored the salmon fisheries. The two CNAs listened intently. Then, Rose said to the legislator, "Sir, you should know about Emily." And she looked at Annette, who shifted in her chair, leaned forward, and with utter sincerity, Rose said, "Sir, I take good care of Emily. A nicer woman you will not find. All her life she has given to her kids and to her foster kids. She is eighty-nine. Alzheimer's has stolen her mind. Emily is so afraid of the dark that she panics when she shuts her eyes. She thinks she is there alone in the pitch-dark night. So I make it a point to get in bed with her, and I sing to her till she drifts into sleep. Now, sir, please think what your vote will do to Emily. My hours will be cut, I won't be able to sing to Emily, and this good woman will spend many a nightmarish night."

The nursing homes were spared this round of cuts.

What Rose and Annette did is a small strand in a mighty tale of a rare and daring venture to empower sixty-four thousand CNAs—caregivers at the bottom of the health-care pecking order. That endeavor was the brainchild of Mary Tellis-Nayak. (*Note: My [VT-N's] credentials to narrate this story are impeccable. Mary is my spouse; we are partners in all our professional undertakings. And she wants me tell you what happened.*)

After much reflection, Mary had accepted the position as the head nurse and chief clinician of a publicly traded large nursing home chain. Her winning ways earned her the confidence of the big boys at the helm. On her recommendation, the company hired the charismatic Bethany Knight as a help to Mary. Knight was a woman with an unfettered imagination and affection for CNAs. Soon, Lori Porter, CEO and founder of the National Association of Health Care Assistants, joined them as a consultant.

This formidable troika cooked up a daring scheme. They were focused on CNAs in the company's five-hundred-plus nursing homes.

The CNAs provided 80 percent of the personal care and yet possessed much untapped potential; they had insights into improving care, eliminating inefficiencies, reducing waste, and calming families. Some had street smarts and uncanny wisdom about human behavior; some were born leaders with no clue of their talent.

So Mary set up a Corporate CNA Council (CCC) that would assist her in nurturing a person-centered culture at the grassroots. She chose as allies the twenty-seven group vice presidents (GVPs), each presiding over twenty-two regional nursing homes. Under Mary's guidance, the GVPs set up regional CNA Councils (CCs). The CCC and the regional CCs had a representation in all corporate committees, whose responsibilities affected the work of the CNAs: purchasing, scheduling, and care planning.

Wisely Mary guided them to choose the first task: to ease the financial squeeze in their nursing home caused by the changed reimbursement in therapy. The CCs came up with an impressive list of money savers. Under the slogan "An empty room is a dark room," everyone went about turning lights off in empty conference rooms, switching off idling computers and unused devices. Kleenex boxes and such were no longer placed right above the toilet to prevent them from accidentally falling in the toilet bowl. Color printing was no longer the default option. One-sided printed paper was recycled and used again.

In one notable case, a CC wrote to the manufacturer of the gloves in Malaysia, suggesting they pack the gloves in the dispenser box so that when you pulled out one glove, two or more did not pop out and had to be discarded. The manufacturer thanked the CNAs and promised that the next shipment would have more intelligently packed boxes of gloves.

These and other victories reverberated through the company and triggered an avalanche. Mary's bosses reaffirmed their support. Twenty-three of the twenty-seven GVPs (regional group VPs) lined up for Mary's team to open CCs for their regions. By year's end, twenty-four fully functioning CCs were chugging ahead full steam with a trail of 516 nursing homes.

Mary's team quickly drew up an ambitious agenda. They coached the CCs on the best way to stay connected and to advance in a coordinated strategy. That blueprint covered performance improvement, ongoing education, and exercising leadership—which led Rose and Annette to identify legislator JW as the crucial vote on budget cuts; they lobbied successfully and won. Other CNAs showed up in other state capitols and drew attention to their cause in quirky tactics, like offering homemade cookies to get lawmakers to listen to them. In one case, a lawmaker was shaken, incredulous, and at a loss for words after hearing a CNA tell him she spent a half hour of wages just to buy milk for her infant.

Mary, a public speaker of note, asked some CNAs to copresent with her when she addressed professional groups. At an AMDA convention attended by medical directors of nursing homes, Alicia, a budding leader in the CCC, spoke on doctor-CNA relations. Alicia rose to the occasion and spoke with such poise and so movingly that the audience of one-hundred-plus doctors gave her a prolonged standing ovation.

In advancing the agenda, CNAs simplified the language and content of routine forms; they pointed out redundancies, overlap, and inconsistencies in policies, procedures, and protocols. In short, the CCs proved to be a source of efficiencies, insights, and unexplored possibilities.

Mary showcased the CCs' success, both within the company and without. The CC members and their accomplishments were recognized and celebrated. With a little prodding from Mary, vendors to the company extended to the CNAs discounted prices for purchases of household supplies and personal care products. Every ten months, representatives from the CCs met for a retreat held at a modest but personable resort. During the three learn-and-relax days, they met with their company associates from different corners of the country. They took stock of their successes and missteps; they kept abreast of the latest developments in their field; they got to know Mary, Bethany, and Lori at a personal level; and they mingled with the president of the company, who went to address them.

However, it was not all smooth sailing. Two GVPs became upset due to their perception that the CCs favored the CNAs over the nurses. The two GVPs did not install CCs in their nursing homes. The old-style administrators and DONs in a few nursing homes viewed these empowered CNAs as upstarts. A few bluntly told them: "Now, don't you get a puffed head. Remember, you are just an aide in this facility." Mary had not anticipated this kink: some CNAs had never been inside an airplane; now they had to learn the new culture of the friendly skies.

Mary received, and continues to receive, e-mails and handwritten cards from CNAs, saying how beholden they feel to her for making them believe in themselves, for helping them to discover their hidden talent, and for making them new people.

Mary had hoped for such transformation but had not thought much about its unexpected consequences. CNAs who grew to be leaders, mentors, and achievers found it hard to survive under authoritarian and disrespectful managers. Their new horizons promised them adventure beyond the CNA role, so some left. On a personal level, a CNA from an eastern state who had approached Mary for guidance regarding the sorry conditions of her marriage—her brutish husband had once locked her in the trunk of his car—thanked Mary and the CCs in a long letter for the courage they gave her to move out of her nightmarish marriage.

The adventure of the CCs illustrates how the themes of humanity, self-identity, empowerment, and self-actualization play out on the floors of nursing homes. That CCs came into being and operated successfully in the very backyard of Wall Street is a feat of leadership that will grace the annals of long-term care.

But Wall Street won. A new CEO, schooled in its ways, came to reign over the company. Soon, he ordered rounds of cuts. Mary was let go in the first round. They gave her no chance to bid good-bye to any of the thousands of CNA friends she left behind.

Climate Conducive for Self-Actualization

A study in 2007 addressed this issue (10.04). The study was massive in scope. The data included responses from 3,579 CNAs and 6,502 families of residents from 156 nursing homes. It added to this data the state inspection survey data for the same nursing homes.

Given the large number of variables and the huge scope of the study, the analysis yielded many findings and insights. We highlight a few that are pertinent to our discussion.

- How well managers listen and care for the CNAs determine how satisfied, loyal, and committed CNAs are in a nursing home.
- CNAs judge their managers exactly the way they assess their workplace. That is, CNAs consider their workplace the truest measure of how much the managers value them as persons.
- Person-centered managers fit a pattern. A manager who respects the CNA as a person empathizes with her difficulties at work and her troubles at home, shields her from difficult residents and demanding families, makes work challenging and less burdensome, delegates, and empowers the CNA and applauds her success. Such a humane manager appeals to the CNA's humanity, stirs her noblest

instincts, motivates her to reach for excellence, to be her best, and to self-actualize.

- Wages are not a CNAs strongest motivator; the attitude of managers and supervisors are.
- Caring managers clone caring supervisors. CNA loyalty increases when supervisors care about them as persons, but only when the managers also do.
- By far, the CNAs' greatest satisfaction comes from knowing that they make a difference in the lives of the residents they care for.

This and similar studies show that the human yearning for self-actualization and for a meaningful life is as strongly evident among the lowest-ranked workers as it is among those socially most privileged. The desire to spread one's wings, to create, and to contribute is an equal opportunity, universal human urge that cuts across all social distinctions. Material incentives and a higher wage will not buy a CNA's commitment. Her deepest satisfaction is her reward for the compassion with which she cares for the residents.

Thus, the need to self-actualize, to reach our ideal self, and to have purpose in life—that need is inherent in the patient and doctor, in the worker and the manager, in the CNA as well as the CEO. Every one yearns to grow, to self-actualize. Everyone has the right to have the room to be all that one can.

Part 2. Humans' Search for Meaning

On April 17, 1945, American forces entered Hitler's concentration camps. Among the liberated was prisoner number 119,104, Viktor Frankl, the towering scholar, researcher, and teacher who opened new doors in positive psychology. Modern-day stress, frustration, and mental illness, he argued, are inevitable when one has no meaning and purpose in life (10.05). He had reached this conclusion through his extensive work with women prone to suicide. That idea led to a momentous discovery when he was a victim of, and witness to, the incredible brutality in Hitler's camp. Frankl's scientific curiosity unearthed one remarkable human trait. Although he and his fellow prisoners suffered the same dire circumstances, Frankl could predict who among them would succumb and who would triumph and survive.

Careful observation and reasoning led him to conclude that even in the most absurd, painful, and dehumanized situation, human life has meaning; you triumph over suffering when you find meaning in suffering. Search for the meaning of life, and happiness will follow when you have discovered it.

From birth we long for fulfillment; we wish to live a life with purpose. This quest is so distinctively human that nature has tied that longing directly to our general well-being. The Center for Disease Control tells us that about four out of ten Americans have not discovered a satisfying life purpose (10.06). About 40 percent do not think they have a clear sense of purpose or cannot say they have. Almost 2 million deaths a year result from top ten causes. This means, at least 1.2 million deaths per year are likely to be affected by a lack of meaning and purpose in life. Those who lack meaning in their lives face a 23 percent greater risk of death and a 19 percent greater risk of death related to the heart. A review of ten studies involving more than 137,000 people found that the people who felt fulfilled suffered fewer strokes and heart attacks and needed fewer surgeries for artery bypass cardiac stents (10.07). Multiple studies have found senior citizens are less likely to face Alzheimer's and late-age ill health when they maintain a sense of purpose.

Frankl narrated an anecdote about finding meaning in suffering:

"Once, an elderly general practitioner consulted me because of his severe depression. He could not overcome the loss of his wife who had died two years before and whom he had loved above all else. Now how could I help him? What should I tell him? I refrained from telling him anything, but instead confronted him with a question, 'What would have happened, Doctor, if you had died first, and your wife would have had to survive you?' 'Oh,' he said, 'for her this would have been terrible; how she would have suffered!' Whereupon I replied, 'You see, Doctor, such a suffering has been spared her, and it is you who have spared her this suffering; but now, you have to pay for it by surviving and mourning her.' He said no word but shook my hand and calmly left the office" (10.08).

When there is no way out, there is always a way through. Perspective gives meaning to illness; clutter falls away, and we see what it means to be alive. We are more fully alive than ever before. Death teaches about life.

One blogger writes, "While I wish I didn't have to get cancer to find out, this is the best thing that's ever happened to me. It helped me to heal my life. It's pushed me to find myself. It all makes sense to me now. And I am at peace with it all" (10.09).

And another, "Cancer taught me to walk through the things I'm afraid of, to let love into the scary places, to be open to experiences that dance on the edge of life. These teachings stay with me. I cherish them. I alternate between feeling frustrated I have to do this again, hopeful that it won't be hideous, and in this wildly open, adventurous place. This is sacred fire that warms me, that lights my path. I know I can go where I need to, spiritually, physically. And I want to. Don't pray to make it easy. Pray for the presence to be truly whole" (10.10).

Illness is a teacher. But you find scant reference to it in medical textbooks. A typical doctor does not primarily see herself or himself as a teacher and often ignores the redemptive meaning of pain—it can open a window to self-knowledge, new possibilities, and a new direction to life.

The yearning for fulfillment and meaning assumes greater significance when we face death. Many have noted that the bureaucratic culture of a hospital, the inhumane ways of managed care, and sterile protocols rob the last days of our life on this earth of fulfillment, satisfaction, meaning, and purpose.

The Culture of Modern Dying

The CDC reports that the proportion of those dying in hospitals declined from nearly half in 1989 to a third in 2007, the proportion of deaths at home increased from 15 percent in 1989 to 24 percent in 2007, and the proportion of deaths in nursing homes rose from 16 percent in 1989 to 22 percent in 2007. That is, over half of American deaths occur within an institutional culture of death not conducive to dying in dignity (10.11).

As death becomes near, some concerns become salient: matters of the spirit, purpose of life, questions about self-worth, self-identity, reconciliation, forgiveness, and compassion. Sharon Kaufman conducted an ethnographic study of dying in a hospital (10.12). She illuminated the complexity of the care dying patients get in hospitals. Slogans such as "Death with dignity," "Quality of life," and "Stopping life support" get muddied amid the idiosyncrasies of hospital life. The rush and pressure around a dying patient obscure the real needs and wishes of the patient. They place the anxious family in the fog between decision and indecision. They make it probable that we will die precisely the way we feared we would and wished we would not. Hospital bureaucracy orphans decision making, diffuses accountability, and manipulates death.

Sometimes the doctors cloud the issue and confuse values. Oncology nurse Theresa Brown wrote in the *New York Times* about her elderly patient who had beaten the odds and lived for ten more years (10.13). But then his lymphoma finally got the better of him. He could no longer say what he wanted, so his wife and son, sad but clear-eyed, chose to stop all treatment and move him to hospice care.

"Hearing this, his oncologist, standing beside me at the nurse's station, cried, heartbroken that her patient of so many years would not rally one more time," Brown wrote. That evening, the patient's primary care doctor came and decided there was hope yet; the patient needed rehab to make him strong enough for more chemotherapy. The oncologist was relieved with the move from hospice to rehab. Soon after the move, the patient died. Brown concluded, "And this was far from the first time I've seen something like this happen"

Anthony Cirrillo, a health-care consultant, spoke about the last days of his father-in-law, Lou (10.14).

"Lou was hospitalized and never made it home. While 51 days of his hospital experience were miserable, the last day of his life was peaceful and dignified. His last day was spent in hospice in the hospital through a separate company not affiliated with the hospital. The culture difference was glaring. And hospice workers were truly caring.

"First, they respected the family's wishes. I married into a large Irish family, and there were probably twenty of us around his bed as they withdrew support. Even a cousin from Northern Ireland, a priest, came over and administered last rites. The hospice nurse simply let us have our space while she explained necessary information in a respectful manner.

"As we moved my father-in-law into a private room, the hospice aide respectfully stayed in the shadows. As one hour led to two, it was clear that my father-in-law was waiting for something before he left us. The hospice nurse suggested that he might not pass with that many people around, especially with his devoted wife of sixty-four years in the room. We took that as a sign to start taking shifts, and my wife, her sister, her niece, and I kept vigil as others went home to get something to eat.

"Obviously, hospice knows a thing or two about dying, because less than an hour after most people left, Lou passed away. It was peaceful—I've never been present when someone died. The aide came in, and once the death was verified, she took the most loving care of this man whom she did not know. She shaved him and bathed him. But it is hard to describe the love she showed while doing it. I watched, probably more so than my grieving wife and her sister.

"But for sporadic episodes, Lou's hospital care was nothing like his care at death. Sure, there were some caring staff. And there were others in and out just doing their job. But the experience was more than staff. The environment reflected it. He spent fifty-one days in a room that my wife and her sisters felt compelled to clean. He stared at a ceiling vent that was dirty, which my sister-in-law eventually cleaned. Were it not for his family advocating for his care, he might have died months before.

"I observed a complete breakdown in communication. No one seemed to know what the others were doing. That was reflected in his two readmissions to the same hospital prior to the last and final visit. It persisted to the last day, when the renal doctor came in to say they would be trying dialysis again, even while the family's wishes of withdrawing support were documented days before."

In recent years, hospitals and nursing homes have intensified a practice that disrespects choice of dying patients and robs them of a dignified, peaceful death. Increasingly, they shuttle persons from home to hospital to nursing home and back again during the last days and weeks of their lives. One study found that, of those residents with advanced cognitive impairment that died in nursing homes between 2000 and 2007, one in four suffered at least one burdensome transition, many in three days before death (10.15). Such relocations add stress increase risk of medical error.

Models and Exemplars of Palliative Care: The Carmelite Path

The spirit of charity that burned brightly on Mount Carmel in days long past also inspired saints through the ages and radiates today in the lives and work of the Catholic Carmelite nuns. These women have dedicated their life to serve poor elderly. Overwhelmingly they are engaged in giving hands-on care to the elders. But some, like Sister Peter Lilian, push the elder cause on the level of policy and education. Sr. Peter Lilian heads the Carmelite Avila Institute of Gerontology (10.16). The institute currently is all geared up to enrich the concept and practice of palliative care by infusing it with the Carmelite spirit.

The aim of palliative care is to relieve pain and to bring comfort to persons with disability of age or illness. Often it is associated with hospice care, and in a medicalized health-care culture, it leans too much on curative intervention. The Avila Institute's objective is to restore balance within palliative care, to reinforce a holistic approach, and to enhance the quality of the patient's last days of life.

One telling detail from one Carmelite nursing home gives a glimpse into the Carmelite reverence for life. A resident had just passed amid hushed prayers, and the body was readied with due respect and dignity. As the procession with the body began to move toward the front door, a musical alert chimed through the nursing home and beckoned the staff throughout the home to observe a minute of silence and prayer. The caregivers who served the deceased resident joined family and mourners, stepped forward, and placed a white rose on the draped body.

The Avila approach professes:

1. Palliative care should address not only the physical but also the existential and spiritual deficits and pain of patients. Those shortcomings need correction.
2. Palliative care should complement its pharmaceutical solutions for pain with helping clients seek meaning in suffering and pain.
3. Palliative care conducts client assessment using sterile quantitative measures lacking in depth and context; it should rely more on qualitative ethnographic, multidisciplinary, and historical and biographical methodologies.
4. Staff training should teach empathy, elements of ethnography and skills of participant observation, grammar of body language, and the art of therapeutic interviews.
5. The training and practice should include educational materials that promote the Carmelite approach to palliative care and tools appropriate to guide its practice.

Part 3. Nuggets of Compassion

Despite the epidemic of the dehumanizing virus, human compassion survives and never ceases to inspire. End-of-life care has expanded vigorously. Hospice and palliative care bring comfort and dignity to the dying. The Butterflies Are Free program, profiled below, is an exemplary model created by an exemplar of compassion, Nina Willingham. The following are but a few blossoms from this garden of compassion and love cultivated by Nina Willingham and other pioneers.

Butterflies Are Free

Nina Willingham (NW) is a leader par excellence who hides her extraordinary people skills behind the quiet efficiency that you notice in the nursing home she runs, Life Care Centers of Sarasota. But you cannot hide excellence under a bushel basket. Her nursing home brims over with trophies and awards it has earned under Nina's leadership: it is listed among America's top nursing homes year after year, it is voted as Life Care Centers of America Facility of the Year, it won The Joint Commission's Ernest A. Codman Award, it won the *Nursing Home Magazine*'s OPTIMA Award, and it won AHCA's Gold Award—this only a partial litany.

Always scanning the horizon for new challenges, Nina instinctively fell for the promises of palliative care. Soon, an interdisciplinary team was busy giving concrete shape to Nina's dream project. As you would expect, Nina's team took the rational route toward a compassionate end. First, they studied the issues and assessed the needs of their nursing home; they combed the archives, reviewed the best models around, and rallied enthusiasm and support. Then they designed a program they called Butterflies Are Free.

The meticulous planning did not miss a detail. The program blends smoothly with the rhythm and flow of the life in the nursing home. It encourages all staff to contribute and families to participate. It incorporates every element that makes such an initiative effective, every process that ensures its success and many heartwarming flourishes that set it apart as excellent.

One of these profoundly simple expressions of compassion is the Butterfly journal. This is an elegantly laid out, handsomely bound journal. You find it in each of the dying patient's room. It invites staff, visitors, or family to record their personal reflections and sentiments. One CNA entry said, "Joe, I stopped in to see you, but you were asleep, resting comfortably." Another entry said, "Sarah, I love our little visits when you tell me about your daughters and how much they mean to you." When the resident passes, all staff take time to write and tell the family what their dear one meant to them. Nina never misses adding a few words of appreciation to the family for their help, friendship, and example.

When the resident passes, Nina gives the family a beautiful keepsake box with the Butterfly journal and a copy of the book *Beyond This Day*—that helps families during their days of grief.

Butterflies Are Free is a shining model and a teacher. It inspires and teaches you how to felicitously translate into everyday practice the lofty principles of compassion, self-actualization, a purposeful life, and a meaningful death. We offer a few more nuggets from this program at the end of this chapter.

Music Resurrects Joe

Joe, a burly Irishman, a gentle, lovable patriarch and a doting father of two professional women, is nearing death. A cruel disease has ravaged his brain and flipped his personality 180 degrees. He does not recognize his daughters; he hurls ugly, hurtful words at them. Each visit devastates them; the foul-mouthed stranger is definitely not their father, who was better than the best of fathers.

The care conferences explored every way to reach the real Joe. Then, the nurse asked about Joe's favorite music. That turned on the light in youngest daughter Margaret's mind. Wide-eyed, she said, "We have some cassette tapes of Daddy singing his Irish songs for us when we were little girls. Would that work?"

It was Joe's last day. His daughters stood each on either side of his bed. He was not able to communicate. Margaret placed the cassette tape in the player, and Joe's beautiful voice filled the air. It took only minutes. Joe's eyes opened, and Joe sang, mouthing the words with obvious relish. He recognized his daughters; to each he said, "I love you"— words they had not heard from their father in years.

At Joe's funeral, the two sisters stood together at the pulpit and told the story of their father's musical resurrection.

Minnie's Final Dance

Minnie was an accomplished young ballerina. But then Myasthenia Gravis cruelly paralyzed her feet, worked its way up her body, paralyzing her, strangling her vocal cords, and then robbing her of the ability to breathe.

At NW's nursing home, Minnie quickly became everyone's favorite. She always had a smile for you and a kind word or gesture for her caregivers.

On the day they thought was Minnie's final day on earth, Debbie, the DON, wanted to thank Minnie in a special way and to alert heaven that Minnie was on her way home.

Minnie loved the sun, so Debbie turned Minnie's bed to face the window, allowing the sun to light up her face. Debbie played beautiful classical music for Minnie's last dance. When the music swelled, Debbie would say, "Oh, Minnie, you just jumped into his arms… He is lifting you high. You are such a beautiful ballerina." In step with the music, Debbie would compliment Minnie as she stretched, bent, rose up, leaped, darted, and glided. Debbie talked to Minnie through the entire dance. The staff showed up, lined up around her bed, holding her hand, touching her forehead, and loving her as she had loved them.

Minnie died peacefully later that day. And everyone knew that Minnie had danced her way into heaven on her own toes, feet, and legs.

Corrie's Broom Sweeps Guilt Away

Petite Corrie, a ninety-one-year-old resident at NW's nursing home, suffered a severe stroke and was in a coma. Her daughter flew out from California. She had always bemoaned that she came only twice a year from California, while her sister lived in the neighborhood and could be with Mama whenever she wished.

A CNA wheeled into the Butterfly room a Butterfly cart carrying toiletries, essential oils, accessories, and books suited for different ages and needs of a grieving family. The CNA found Sue, the California daughter, sobbing by the bed of her mother, who lay unconscious. Sue admitted that she felt guilty being unable to do much for her mother. The empathetic CNA suggested that she sit with her sister by her mother and exchange childhood memories. "Your mother may hear your voices and feel happy with your stories."

Soon the two daughters and their husbands were seated close to Mama and, sotto voce, were reconstructing their life with their mother as they took turns rubbing her back and anointing her with fragrant oils. As soft music played, the stories continued. Sue said to the mother, "Mama, I remember how you used to chase us around the kitchen table with a broom until you caught us, and then you swatted us on our behinds until we promised to be better." The husbands added details. Soon, smiles turned to laughter and laughter to hearty guffaws that resounded down the hallways. The laughter was therapy. It purged irrational regrets and guilt and gave them a reason to celebrate the glorious motherly feats of Corrie.

They were sure their mother met her creator with a chuckle on her face and laughter in her heart.

CHAPTER 11

The Human Need and Right to Reach Beyond

I slept and I dreamed that life is all joy.
I woke and I saw that life is all service.
I served and I saw that service is joy.
—*Kahlil Gibran*

Part 1. Exercise Your Heart

You hear it said, "There is no exercise better for the heart than reaching down and lifting people up." That is literally true. Deep within us lurks a primal yearning to break out of selfishness and to serve others. Nature has hardwired us with tendencies toward kindness, generosity, forgiveness, and self-sacrifice. These tendencies help us achieve the goals of evolution—namely, survival, gene replication, and easy coexistence of groups. In this chapter, we will look at the curious ways in which altruism interfaces with health care. We will look at the quality of generosity, when it is merely a self-serving ruse and when it is a deeply human gesture that cures, fortifies the spirit, and gives meaning to life and dignity to death.

Dacher Keltner, director of the Berkeley Social Interaction Laboratory, investigates these matters in *Born to Be Good: The Science of a Meaningful Life.* Forget survival of the fittest, he argues, it is kindness that counts; kindness is the instinct for self-preservation (11.01).

Darwin did not portray humans as violent, competitive, and self-interested. Survival of the fittest was not what Darwin said; that was the slogan used by Herbert Spencer and social Darwinists to justify social inequality. Darwin argued that "communities with the greatest number of sympathetic members would flourish best, and rear the greatest number of offspring." Compassion indeed is a naturally evolved adaptive trait that has ensured the survival of our species. No wonder men and women consider compassion and kindness as the most highly valued traits in romantic partners. In teasing and provocative play, researchers note, coyotes that bite too hard are relegated to low-status positions.

Keltner points to the physiological underpinning of compassion. Connecting with others meaningfully leads to better mental and physical health, speeds up recovery from disease, and lengthens our life span. Giving is more pleasurable than receiving. The pleasure centers in the brain that are activated during dessert and sex also become active when we observe someone giving money to charity. Giving to others increases pleasure more than when receiving. In one experimental study published in science, participants who had spent money on others felt significantly happier than those who had spent money on themselves. This is true even for infants. In children as young as two years old, giving treats to others increases the giver's happiness more than receiving treats themselves. Even more surprisingly, the fact that giving makes us happier than receiving is true across the world, regardless of whether countries are rich or poor.

Activation of the vagus nerve affects feelings of compassion. A new science of happiness is finding that compassion and kindness can be readily cultivated in familiar ways, bringing out the good in others and in oneself.

Transcendence in Health Care

On a sunny spring day—the specific date is lost to history—at Mission View Health Center, a nursing home in San Luis Obispo, California, administrator Matthew Lysobey was listening intently to his staff as they pondered the question he posed to them: "We give our residents very good care. We have compassionate, caring staff. Residents tell us they are truly satisfied. Why, then, do they not look happy?" He turned to Sophie, a CNA who, in simple words but with shrewd insight, precisely spelled out the correct diagnosis. "Indeed, we love our residents and serve them with devotion," said Sophie. "That is where the problem may lie. My life would suck if all I had to look forward to every day was thanking everyone for helping me and no one thanked me, because no one needs me anymore."

Elders Reach Out

Sophie's insight into the human heart echoed the conclusions Frankl articulated in his landmark book *Man's Search for Meaning*. The suicidal cases he treated convinced him that suicide is a failure to make sense of life. Ample evidence supports that view. Of the thirty-five thousand suicides annually in the United States, significantly more occur on Mondays, while much fewer happen on holidays; the suicide rate spikes after age sixty-five, but it drops among those who have friends, and it drops even more among those with many friends and close ties (11.02). These findings hint at the power of the spiritual element in human life, its potential to kill or to heal; it can lift us out of our self-absorption and help us transcend, to reach out and to make a difference in others' lives—a sure way to enrich our own life and add joy to it.

The wisdom in Sophie's simple words was born of a CNA's everyday experiences. A CNA has a difficult mandate. The repetitive job routine, the negative public image of her or his workplace, the lowest status position she or he occupies in it, and the meager wages she or he earns all combine to make a CNA's mandate more burdensome. Nevertheless, CNAs are not an alienated lot.

On the contrary, My InnerView/National Research annual surveys of more than four thousand nursing homes show that much of the turnover in their ranks is just a recycling of the same group at the fringes of a solid, stable core (11.03). Nationwide, more than half of all CNAs have worked in the same nursing home for more than a year, and more than 25 percent have worked there for five years or more. MIV also discovered that CNAs' greatest satisfaction comes from making a difference in the lives of those they care for. Altruism, generosity, and transcendence are alive and well among CNAs, although researchers seem blind to it.

The Handicapped Help the Homeless

Lysobey took Sophie's message to heart; he set the stage for the implementation of Helping Hands, a service program dedicated to feeding the homeless once a month. The buy-in was immediate and wide-ranging. Residents, their families, and staff now had a shared mission. They rallied around it, bent their energies, and marshaled every resource toward furthering the cause. They formed think tanks and worked in teams; they assessed needs, planned, and organized. In the process, they unearthed a treasure trove of talent, skills, and experience that lay unseen and unused among the 130 residents, who in their greener years were accomplished engineers, salesmen, teachers, lawyers, and homemakers. That reservoir of expertise would be theirs to tap. In other words, Mission View became a different community, stirred by a lofty vision, abuzz with new energy, with everyone looking in the same direction and anxious to move forward.

Helping Hands' members decided to raise money by making scented homemade soaps to sell at the local farmers' market. The team reviewed the steps they needed to take to make this venture successful and matched the tasks to each resident's expertise: bookkeeping, sales, marketing, publicity, packaging, transport, scheduling—even residents with dementia happily pasted labels on the product.

Over the past several years, Helping Hands has matured into a well-oiled, resident-managed company that has never taken a loan, never failed to pay a bill, never slipped in its schedule, and never turned away a hungry homeless person. The local town takes pride that wheelchairs cruise down its sidewalks. The farmers' market has a new magnate, namely, wheelchair-bound residents offer free homemade cookies to attract customers, who along with the cookie also receive a salutary homily on attaining inner joy by feeding homeless children, which they can do indirectly by purchasing soaps.

"The handicapped helping the homeless makes an inspiring sight," says Dennis Conway, the wheelchair-confined resident and VP of sales at Helping Hands.

There is no telling where it may lead. Helping Hands has branched out. Today, residents offer companionship to hospice patients. They are planning to extend aid to Haiti, they make cash awards to national charities, and they have gone global, selling their signature soap product online.

Part 2. Be Human: Face Outward

You have reason to be happy when your life has meaning and purpose. Your life attains meaning when what you do has value. Nothing is more valuable than pursuing a cause larger than yourself. As Frankl explained, being human always means that you face outward to something or someone other than yourself. The more you forget yourself—by giving yourself to a cause or to a person—the more human you are.

The pursuit of meaning is what makes us uniquely human. By putting aside selfish interests, by *giving* rather than *taking*, you attain the good life and happiness. Frankl recalled, "We who lived in concentration camps can remember the men who walked through the huts comforting others, giving away their last piece of bread. They may have been few in number, but they offer sufficient proof that everything can be taken from a man but one thing: the last of human freedoms—to choose one's own attitude in any given set of circumstances—to choose one's own way" (11.04).

Selfless and Selfish Altruism

Some have argued that, strictly speaking, the services doctors and other clinical practitioners provide cannot be called altruism. We pointed out in chapter 5 that society has given the medical profession certain privileges and rights—to recruit, train, and monitor professional conduct by the standards the medicine sets—for agreeing to meet the health-care needs of the community. This tacit agreement places a fiduciary obligation on doctors. Altruism is not obligatory. What doctors do may deserve praise. But their professional duty to heal, in itself, is not praiseworthy benevolence.

Everyone, however, knows that doctors go beyond the call of duty. The universal admiration for their altruism through groups like

Doctors Without Borders has promoted benevolence and spawned imitators much beyond medicine (see boxed insert).

A survey in England studied doctors in practice and in training and learned that 74 percent of respondents performed altruistic activity outside their normal working practice, and 83 percent of doctors would dedicate a regular amount of time each year toward altruistic work (11.05).

Similar is the case with patients who have the obligation to collaborate, provide all relevant information, comply with treatment, and generally participate in their own care.

Patients manifest altruism when they allow medical students to treat them, when they take part in research or clinical tests and donate blood, organs, and semen. Altruism implies doing good to others without necessarily expecting reciprocity.

Is it altruism when you stand to gain by generosity toward others? When is generosity not altruism?

There is a vast difference between solipsistic, self-centered generosity and selfless service that gives you the helper's high. The former, at one extreme, is selfishness that takes the guise of charity or donation but in truth expects gratification, social recognition, tax avoidance, or other personal profit. The latter, at the opposite extreme, is transcendence that has prompted heroes, saints, and martyrs to risk life and limb in pursuing a higher cause. Between the two extremes lies a gray zone, where genuine benevolence reaps handsome personal profit.

The Wall Street Journal in 2009 profiled India's Dr. Devi Shetty as the Henry Ford of heart surgery, who uses a factory model for heart hospitals to cut costs, maintain quality, and reap profit (11.06). Headlines around the world featured him as Mother Theresa's cardiac surgeon.

Dr. Shetty's Narayana Health network today has hospitals in sixteen locations in India and an international subsidiary in the Cayman

Islands. It runs the Institute of Cardiac Sciences in Bangalore and a multispecialty hospital in Jaipur. The flagship hospital in Bangalore houses dialysis units and India's largest bone marrow transplant unit, and it conducts liver, kidney, and heart transplants. It performs the largest number of successful pediatric heart surgeries in the world. It runs the largest telemedicine networks in the world.

It performs heart surgeries every day; it transplants livers in babies less than ten kilograms with a 95 percent success rate. It performed the first artificial heart implant in Asia. It runs sixty-one training programs. Its Thrombosis Research Institute is bent on discovering a vaccine to prevent heart attack and, to date, has come up with markers to diagnose heart disease early.

Dr. Shetty works on the simple premise of economies of scale. Huge volumes drive down cost. An average heart surgery costs $1,586—half of what it cost twenty years ago—with the target of $800 ten years from now. This compares with $106,000 and rising at the Cleveland Clinic, a U.S. leader. In 2008, forty-two cardiac surgeons in the Bangalore hospital performed 3,174 cardiac bypass surgeries, more than double the 1,367 the Cleveland Clinic did in the same year. His surgeons operated on 2,777 pediatric patients, more than double the 1,026 surgeries performed at Children's Hospital Boston.

According to Dr. Jack Lewin, chief executive of the American College of Cardiology, Dr. Shetty has used high volumes to improve quality; the large number of patients allows individual doctors to focus on one or two specific types of cardiac surgeries. Dr. Shetty's hospitals show a 1.4 percent mortality rate within thirty days of coronary artery bypass graft surgery compared to an average of 1.9 percent in the United States. Dr. Lewin believes Dr. Shetty's success rates would look even better if he adjusted for risk, because his patients often lack access to even basic health care and suffer from more advanced cardiac disease when they finally come in for surgery.

Doctors Without Borders Inspire Altruism

1. **Bikes Without Borders**
   This is a Canadian nonprofit group that travels the world, distributing bicycles to developing communities.
2. **Astronomers Without Borders**
   They share in order to avert star wars.
3. **Burners Without Borders**
   A small group that travels the world promoting radical self-expression and self-reliance in developing communities.
4. **Chemists Without Borders**
   They bring information to help people access safe water, create sustainable energy, and to deal safely with hazardous chemicals.
5. **Clowns Without Borders**
   San Francisco–based group of jesters, trips, pratfalls, and pogosticks go to refugee camps, conflict zones, and crisis areas all around the world, bringing laughter, circus performances, and big red plastic noses to children who need some levity.
6. **Kangaroo Without Borders**
   This group of math-loving Australians spend their spare time organizing mathematics competitions for young people all around the world.
7. **Geeks Without Borders**
   TFrom its home base in Eugene, Oregon, they collect and distribute used computers and technical tools to orphanages, schools, and other organizations around the world.

8. **Words Without Borders**

A small cadre of literary activists publishes stories written by authors from every race and creed in order to connect wordsmiths with one another and foster a global literary conversation.

9. **Pirates Without Borders**

A loose group that believes in free knowledge, free culture, and free software—and are willing to sail the seven seas of the Internet, pillaging paywalls and pirate patented products.

10. **Monks Without Borders**

This motley team of monks, nuns, priests, rabbis, swamis, imams, and clergy members from all the world's religious traditions travel the world, promoting nonviolence and interfaith cooperation wherever they go.

(Source: Mental Floss, January 27, 2012)

The Kindness of Strangers

Now leave the gray zone, where generosity brings modern medicine to the underprivileged and profit to the do-gooder, and move to the bright-green zone, where generosity transmutes into pure compassion. Consider the following epiphany of compassion.

Delta Flight 15 and its 218 passengers were four and a half hours out of Frankfurt when the captain, Michael Sweeney, came on the PA and said there was a problem with the indicator light and the plane would have to land in Gander, Newfoundland, to get it fixed.

When they landed, out of the window, you could see planes from all over the world lined up, one after the other. At the head of one line was a U.S. Air Force cargo plane.

It was September 11, 2001.

Once parked, the captain came back on and apologized for the ruse; there was nothing wrong with the plane, but there was a national emergency in the United States, and the military was now in charge of U.S. airspace. Everything went deathly quiet. People whipped out their cell phones, but no one could get through.

They sat on the tarmac for twenty-four hours, anxious, shaken, and alone, cut off from the world. Sweeney monitored the BBC from the cockpit and relayed the news: one of the towers of the World Trade Center had been hit, the Pentagon had been hit, and something had happened outside of Pittsburgh.

Thirty-eight planes and 8,000 passengers were detoured to Gander and the surrounding area. Passengers of flight 15 and three others were bused to Lewisporte, a no-stoplight town of 3,800 people, forty-five miles from Gander. The school bus drivers had been on strike; they suspended their strike to drive the stranded passengers. Locals came on the bus and told the travelers, "Please don't hesitate. Anything you need, just let us know."

And they had literally thought of everything. When Lewisporte mayor Bill Hooper commandeered the local airwaves to plead for food, blankets, and pillows, people brought in much more: shampoo, diapers, books, toys, baby food, towels, TVs. People hung American flags and flew them at half-mast. Bill Hooper had arranged for TVs and phone banks with no fee or restriction on where to call or how long to talk.

Hooper told the refugees, "We have a feeling in our hearts that you aren't strangers. We are more than happy to be able to be there in your time of desperate need."

But they were more than just there. Some of the passengers had packed their prescription medication in their luggage. So the people in Lewisporte drove them to doctors and then to pharmacists, who filled the prescriptions for free. Women took towels and washcloths home, washed and dried them, and brought them back. Those who cooked never went home although their legs swelled from standing up for so long. The town was essentially closed, and the few shops that were open would not let anyone pay.

This went on for three days. People gave them everything—absolutely everything. It was an exquisite and sublime display of transcendence.

Then the passengers once again sat shoulder to shoulder on the jumbo jet bound for Atlanta. By the time flight 15 touched down, they had pledged the seed money needed to start the Gander Flight 15 Scholarship Fund. Soon, more than $3 million came in as donations to offer scholarships to students in the Lewisporte Collegiate.

A telling case of survival of the kindest.

Part 3. Random Acts of Kindness

The following are a few apparitions of compassion in unexpected places and contexts in health care.

Pillow Talk

After two decades as nurse, Anna still tears up seeing children requiring surgery. Anna had learned to sew. She gave pillowcases as presents and earned the name as the pillowcase maker. She gave a few to the surgery center in the UC Davis Children's Hospital, California. She was surprised; the pillowcases proved a big hit.

When her daughter needed a high school community service project, they decided on a coordinated project. Anna helped purchase precut fabric, and eight needleworkers were busy at work. In three hours, they made 100 pillowcases with prints of princesses, action heroes, and familiar characters that live in childhood fantasies.

The response from nurses, doctors, parents, and patients was overwhelming. "This has changed our world," said one nurse. A child entered the surgery prep area, carrying a stuffed monkey, and found a monkey pillowcase waiting for her on the bed. Parents called to say the pillow reduced their child's anxiety.

Little Tanya hugged her princess pillowcase as she was wheeled out to her family's car. A nurse asked her about princesses and Disneyland. The nurse asked what her favorite part of Disneyland was. Tanya answered, "I don't know, but my favorite part of this day was this pillowcase!"

Pillowcases have a therapeutic effect on mothers. Frustrated mothers see their child smiling and holding tight the pillowcase, and at once, they defuse and even hug the nurse whom they almost cursed a minute ago.

Anna's team has fashioned more than 2,500 pillowcases. Anna hopes to reach 3,000 by year's end. For Anna, it is therapy. "Nursing is stressful. The smiles and stories mean so much to me," she said. A helper from her church sews an average of 20 pillowcases a week and, teary–eyed, said how the pillowcases have added meaning to her life.

The Chrysalis Room

Loretta Downs was distressed seeing that while visitors surround a dying loved one, helpless roommates suffer the sights, sounds, and smells of death and grief. They lie on the other side of the flimsy curtain where the dead body of your roommate lies alone, awaiting removal.

At Fairmont Care Center, where her mother was a hospice resident, Loretta created a beautifully set Chrysalis Room and moved her in along with her favorite possessions. "The night before she died, half a dozen residents wheeled into the Chrysalis Room to say a rosary, to demonstrate their love for her, and to comfort me while we awaited her transition. Two of my friends came with love and food. I spent the night and was at my mother's side when she died, peacefully, with the morning sun streaming across her bed through white wood blinds.

"We bathed mother's body, dressed her in her favorite robe, covered the bed with flower petals, and invited her resident friends and caring staff to say good-bye. Five hours later, she was escorted out of the building with an honor guard of people who were important to her. I felt proud that I had honored my mother for giving me life by giving her a good death.

"Two of the residents who shared the experience of mother's death told me they want to move to the Chrysalis Room when 'It's my time.'"

Impressed by its success, the Lancaster Corporation, which owns the Fairmont Care Center, has installed Chrysalis Rooms in four of their other nursing homes.

"My dream is to have a Chrysalis Room in every nursing home in America," said Loretta Downs.

The Threshold Choir

Groups of singers from different backgrounds bring ease and comfort to those at the thresholds of living and dying. Their calm presence, gentle voices, simple songs, and genuine kindness soothe and reassure clients, family, and caregivers alike.

When invited, two to four singers go to the bedside. They invite families and caregivers to join in song. They choose songs that are in keeping with the client's musical taste, spiritual leanings, and other needs. The Threshold Choir sings songs, many of which they created, that appeal to general spiritual rather than specific religious life. They sing for about twenty minutes and longer when requested. They sing in soft, lullaby voices, in harmony or in unison—always to provide the most comfort. Their songs convey gentle blessings and do not aim to entertain. When they lull the client into slumber, the singers feel rewarded. Families often continue to sing for their loved one after the Threshold Choir leaves.

The service is a gift from the Threshold Choir. There is no charge.

Kate Munger first assembled the Threshold Choir on the vernal equinox, March 21, 2000, in Katharine Osburn's home in El Cerrito, California. Most of the fifteen women who sang that evening continue to sing in the choir today. Over a hundred Threshold Choir chapters in the United States, Canada, United Kingdom, and Australia add comfort, joy, and meaning to the dying in their last days on earth.

CONCLUSION
Imagine Compassion

"We are all in the gutter, but some of us are looking at the stars."
—*Oscar Wilde*

Part 1. The Lost Art of Healing

Bernard Lown M.D., inventor of the heart fibrillator, and winner of the Nobel Prize is a strong advocate of compassion in health care. Born in Lithuania, he migrated to the U.S. at age 13; he earned his M.D. at Johns Hopkins and went on to become Professor of Cardiology at the Harvard School of Public Health. He narrates an instructive story (C: 1).

A middle-aged man had sought relief from intermittent severe heart arrhythmia. He had visited all the renowned clinical centers and had received no credible diagnosis and treatment. He ended up in the office of Dr. Lown. As wont, Dr. Lown began by probing the patient's background and history." How many grand kids do you have?" At once, the room fell silent; gears shifted; the tone changed. The patient became uncomfortable; he gazed down and studied the floor. "Do you have any grand kids?" Now, the patient looked up teary eyed: "Yes, four."

Dr. Lown soon learned why the patient was agitated. He had an altercation with his son on a business matter that concluded with his son yelling at him: "You will never see your grandkids again!" That was ten years ago, the years that he had been bothered by his heart condition. He suffered a devastating blow to his ego, to his legacy and to his yearning for family. It affected his body; it left scars in his mind and pain in his heart. Dr. Lown set him on the road to recovery.

He thanked the doctor profusely. Dr. Lown never saw him again (12.01).

Dr. Lown goes on to lament "the lost art of healing." The commercialization of human relations, the loss of community and the dehumanization of work have shaken loose many spheres of life from their moorings. Modernity has not spared health care. It has lured health care down a covetous path.

"At what point does it become a crime?" asks H. Gilbert Welch, Professor of medicine at Dartmouth" (C: 2). In Denver, he notes, a patient whose cardiac stress test cost around $2,000 in 2014, and around $8,000 in 2015, after his doctor's practice was bought by the hospital. Medical care is intended to help people, not enrich providers. But it looks less like help than like highway robbery."

In the first quarter of the last century, Abraham Flexner had given medical training a narrow, scientific focus. Towards the end of the century, medicine took a sharp turn on to Market Street, that led it farther away from its person-centered tradition. Regulators imposed market discipline to curb health care's fiscal excesses. Through that opening, a new mind-set invaded health care, like an alien predatory species it spread unchecked. Market thinking aligned with the interests of pharmaceutical and insurance companies. Managed care came to dominate hospital operations, nursing home policies and clinical practice.

The shift from appreciation of value to an obsession with cost has wrought a sea change in the in health care. Doctor-patient trust has soured; angry consumers resort to malpractice suits; doctors view patients as potential enemies. Managed care and regulation have robbed clinicians of their autonomy, of the satisfaction that comes from relationships. Alienation among caregivers has strained personal relationships. These negatives have set the stage for clinical errors and the perpetuating the vicious cycle.

The health care sky is gray and gloomy. But there is a break in the clouds giving us a peek into an alternate world; it is a foretaste of the blessings of compassion we all yearn for and stalwarts dare to anticipate. These exemplars, undeterred and unbowed, have made compassion sprout in its myriad expressions across the length and breadth of health care, in unexpected places and forbidding contexts. They never cease to edify us.

Four themes resonate through these exemplary attempts at putting compassion into action.

The Survival of the Kindest

First, compassion is a divine virtue, yet it is profoundly human. Compassion is one among the five primal urges that nature has etched in our DNA. As the noblest of human traits, compassion spiritualizes us. It lifts us above selfishness and prompts us to sympathize with and share the pain in others.

The science of compassion and altruism has shown that generosity activates the same pleasure-linked brain neurons that are triggered when you enjoy a bar of chocolate. Similar brain activity has been documented in young children when they give and share than when they receive. The same results are repeated across nations and cultures. Evolutionary biologists explain why compassion is so intimately part of our makeup. Altruism gave us an edge in the survival game. Darwin wrote about the "survival of the kindest," not of the fittest. Caring, altruism and compassion served human groups well in especially three crucial situations: a mother's selfless caring of the infant, a lover's concern for the mate, and an individual's loyalty and service to the group.

Our need to transcend selfishness comes bundled with our other basic needs: to be, to become, to belong and to be one's best. They were vital to our evolutionary strategy and they continue to be vital today for our life, health and wellbeing. We think of them as distinct; but in practice, they overlap, form a network and interact. Any trouble in one area can reverberate through the network causing collateral damage to the person's health and wellbeing.

Thus, an ideal clinician pursues symptoms back to its roots. Just two generations ago, clinicians entered practice schooled in the ways of science and well mentored by experienced and wise teachers to tune in to human conduct, its unspoken subtleties, and hidden grammar. They began their diagnostic exploration with a ritual examination of the symptoms. Then with a cultivated instinct, they surveyed the patient's life tracing illness to its hidden roots in the crevices of one's biography, beyond the reach of technology.

Their training also made them internalize their obligation to heal the whole person. Indeed to extend their concern to the suffering family and needy care-givers.

In a person-centered environment, each participant is a patient and a healer; each impacts the other's wellbeing; each has rights as well as obligations to the others. A truly person-centered hospital ensures the patient's recovery, relieves the stress of the family, affirms the autonomy of the clinicians and provides a quality workplace for the support team.

Compassion in a Person-Centered Culture

A second theme runs through the theory and practice of compassion. Compassion awaits awakening in the human heart. In an organization, it multiplies, spreads and flowers in a climate of mutual respect and caring.

Herein lies health care's biggest handicap. Many people of good will launch rationally designed person-directed programs, but disregard an obvious fact of life. Every organization, hospital or nursing home, operates at two levels. At orientation, a newcomer learns the organizational chart, lines of authority and job expectations. These are marks of the formal culture of the organization.

Another informal culture operates parallel to the official culture of an organization. It is the informal culture made up of personal ties, friendly obligations, loyalties, intrigues, power-tugs, favoritism, gossip and rumor. This world runs by its own logic, rules and expectations which you learn on your own as a new employee. The two systems may coexist or work at cross purposes. When guided by a wise manager the two worlds complement each other, coalesce, and become a cultural bulwark of quality and compassion.

A cultural audit would reveal that many health care centers lack an optimal integration even in their official organizational structure. Most people notice the pockets of informal subcultures operating at the workplace, but fail to recognize that informal networks can enhance or thwart official agenda. Their countervailing dynamics or can douse compassionate impulses or defeat person-centered initiatives. When there exists no supportive culture and no benign manager to create it, many a noble venture flickers and flames out. That is, a shared a sense of community and mutual regard is the nourishing climate for compassion to flower.

Humane Leaders Create a Caring Workplace

A third theme relates to the pivotal role of executives in the creation and sustaining of a person-focused culture.

Poor quality in a hospital or care-facility reflects a mediocre leadership. The character and culture of a health care center does not rise above the vision and moral caliber of its manager. A seasoned manager assigned to redeem an unbecoming situation rife with rivalries, colliding egos, and clashing cliques, knows the challenge ahead. It is a challenge to rally the factions around a compelling vision; to stir their noblest instinct to achieve a worthy goal; to help turn themselves into a community where everyone interacts warmly across social roles, treats each other with respect and trust, and shares and collaborates. Indeed the grandest feat of a manager is transforming unengaged workers into a team of caring care-givers.

Teamwork in a complex health care center, like a hospital, is not unlike teamwork on a soccer field, nor is a hospital manager different from a soccer coach. A soccer game features highly skilled and fiercely competitive egos working in graceful harmony towards a common goal. They move in synch in a concerted strategy; they are tuned into each other, they read precisely each other's thoughts, they anticipate each other's move; they improvise, yield, retreat, outwit— all this to reach their shared goal, victory for their team and glory to themselves. The exquisite interplay of mind, muscle, skill, and grace is a tribute to the coach, as it is to the manager, who assembled the talent, mixed, matched and shaped that talent into an unbeatable team—a showcase of effective communication, interdependence, cooperation and collaboration. A triumph brings people together; it helps you to learn about and know others as persons, to appreciate their talent, to share their joy as well as their troubles.

A Sublime Virtue in a Mundane World

The fourth theme touches on a topic that puzzles everyone, but is rarely discussed by anyone. It is natural to expect that compassion, so lofty an ideal, yet so delicate and tender in display, would surely wilt in the withering heat of competition and profit-maximization. Is compassion incompatible with business principles? Is compassion an anomaly in a capitalist society?

The answer is evident, unambiguous and transparently clear. Research and elementary logic bring us to the same conclusion. Compassion, as well as our other virtuous impulses, is not incongruent with our innate drive to seek profit. On the contrary, although seemingly polar opposites, they are two sources of human happiness, two innate tendencies that serve our needs at two different levels.

Many hold that compassion and self-interest are irreconcilable and belong to different and contradictory sectors of life. The marketplace is the battleground where rivals follow the law of the wild to eliminate competitors. Benevolence, service and charity are beatitudes worthy of a Sermon on the Mount.

Adam Smith, the patron saint of economists, had pointed out that the "passion" (the natural human need) towards benevolence was a distinct human trait, but different from "self-interest" and "selfishness." "It is not from the benevolence of the butcher, the brewer, or the baker that we expect our dinner, but from their regard to their own self-interest." Self-interest contributes to the common good. It is complemented by human urge to reach out and help others.

He decried selfishness in personal life and in trade. Greed, avarice, and selfishness are enemies of the free market. Monopolies, price-fixing, insider trading and trade pacts hinder the working of the invisible hand. Adam Smith favored government regulation and intervention to ensure the common good.

His book, *The Theory of Moral Sentiments*, published in 1759, opens with an implicit swipe at Hobbes's egocentrism and with an overt nod to altruism: "How so ever selfish man may be supposed, there are evidently some principles in his nature, which interest him in the fortune of others…they derive nothing from it except the pleasure of seeing it." "The man whom we naturally love the most is he who joins to…his own original and selfish feelings, the most exquisite sensibility…and sympathy he feels for others." Adam Smith elaborates on the "exquisite sensibility and sympathy," generosity, fairness, equality and distributive justice and makes them the building blocks of his theory of human affairs.

Modern articulations of the free market often depart greatly from Adam Smith's theory. For a stark illustration, consider the tycoon or a corporation that lays off workers en masse. They invoke the free market as a fig leaf to hide naked greed. No pangs of conscience disturb their sleep. Terminating workers is rightful "business decision," dictated by the bottom line, an axiom learned in business classes and lauded by Wall Street. Morality and economics are watertight compartments, each with its own code. Thus, business moguls are not morally accountable for the devastation they caused in the lives of the laid-off workers, their families and the communities.

This is yet another case where modernism feeds the baser, selfish human appetites. A valid dualistic philosophy of inquiry now reigns as a dehumanizing ideology; it makes a medic treat the patient as a collection of body parts; it makes an employer look at work and the worker as a commodity.

Adam Smith would have harshly condemned such rationalization that denies the rights of care-givers in nursing homes and hospital. There are shoddy, demeaning practices in the health care workplace that are rationalized with a thin free market gloss.

In the U.S. 68 percent of nursing homes and 18 percent of hospitals, run for for-profit. This makes fiscal viability a paramount consideration. Pursuit of excellence and a person-centered culture make no sense, if they do not make fiscal sense. Abundant research has made a business case for excellence and high quality. A humanitarian path to excellence is good business.

Companies that value their workers and invite employees to be co-owners have better results on various measures of business success—both in health care and outside health care. In long-term care, a good number of nursing homes receive consistently high scores on satisfaction of residents, their families and the care-givers. These care-centers also reap a cornucopia of benefits. Their staff turnover runs low, their no-show or call-in rate is negligibly low. Fewer workers suffer injury which cuts worker compensation costs. Satisfied families pay bills on time, recommend the nursing home to others with more enthusiasm and keep the census high with greater number of private payers and Medicare beneficiaries; excellent care reduces insurance premium, attracts volunteers and donations. Firm evidence shows that revenue per bed correlates the quality in the nursing home.

Part 2. A Call to Health Care Leaders

This overall four-point summary of the developments in person-centered approach projects an image of health care as a wounded Titanic. Market winds impelled it inexorably away from its compassionate moorings into perilous waters. Its captains witnessed the encroachment of the market, but devised no strategy, nor marshaled all their forces to contain its advance, nor shored up the institutional foundations of humane values.

The thousand points of light that keep hope alive are the valiant efforts at re-orienting the health care ship back towards safe harbor. But the land of compassion has not appeared on the horizon.

When will the day of compassion dawn? What can we do to hasten its return?

Many have deployed abundant resources, high expertise and uncommon imagination to remake the workplace and workers into a healing community. We have referenced them; so we will refrain from reciting that litany again.

Instead, we will conclude with a high-minded, yet simple, recommendation. In truth, it is more an appeal than a recommendation. It emerges from an elementary fact of life that we have harped on. In health care, leaders, managers and administrators are the corner stone of sustained quality. Their passion to incarnate a person-focused vision is the best clue to how deeply an organization is wedded to humane care and caring. Our appeal to them is uncomplicated, but we hope for an outsized impact.

We direct our appeal to the following select top leaders in acute and post-acute and long-term care.

- The Board of Trustees, American Hospital Association
- The Board of Commissioners, Joint Commission
- The Board of Trustees, American Medical Association
- The Board of Directors, Association of American Medical Colleges
- The Board of Directors, American Nurses Association
- Board of Governors, National League for Nursing
- The Board of Directors, AMDA – The Society for Post-Acute and Long-Term Care Medicine
- The Board of Governors, American Health Care Association and the Board of Directors, National Center for Assisted Living.
- The Board of Directors, Leading Age

We ask each member of each these Boards, before the end of the next quarter, to take a one-time 30 minute respite from their busy life and devote it to a personal, deep three-part reflection on a life and death issue that we face.

- Begin with a bird's-eye-view mental survey of the health care landscape. Linger on the major wrong turns its leaders took. Before their eyes, health care slid into the quicksand that saps its humanity and human values.

- When medicine let market efficiency bring needed fiscal discipline, it did not intend to open the gates for the market ethos. But the business model soon spread and has come to rule the day. Expediency has eased out sympathy. Productivity and the bottom line have emerged as new measures of success, TQM has fallen by the wayside; excellence and compassion are not the proud symbols in health care. Satisfying Wall Street has become the priority, not patient, family or staff satisfaction.

- Commercialization is now overt, blatant, and at times, even crass. Consumers, angered by high costs, long waits, rushed clinical visits and pervasive clinical errors, resort to malpractice suits, more to punish than for redress. Even in the least sued specialty (pediatricians), 75 percent of doctors, and 99 percent among the most sued (neurosurgeons), will be sued by age 65. Tellingly, the patient wins only one in five cases.

- The unseemly preoccupation with output, work quotas, productivity and profit make a mockery of the practitioner's autonomy, control and freedom. They rob practitioners of the rewards of healing bonds, of the professional challenge new, difficult cases offer. They make the workplace joyless and cause turnover at every level. More than half of all doctors regret the career choice they made; a majority would not recommend doctoring to their children; their divorce rate exceeds the rate among any other profession; they resort to suicide more than professionals in any other group.

- In sum, no one would claim that health care today lives up to its mission to cater to our five primal yearnings. A profession with a mission to promote health does not seem to care for its own. It has made work unrewarding and the work setting joyless and devoid of human warmth.

Now you move on to the second topic for your consideration:

- Reflect on this awesome fact: the formidable power and prestige of the office you occupy as members of the premier governing bodies in health care.
- Skepticism is widespread. But the public looks at you with awe. It correctly thinks of you the best and brightest of your species, learned wise and trustworthy.
- In truth, in health care, you are the axes of power, you have the final word in matters that affect our life, death, health and illness. You can make policy, change training curricula, set standards of practice and codes of behavior. You are at the helm, with ready access to every state-of-the-art tool and resource to do the best for our health and wellbeing.

Now in the last phase, create in your mind a "What if" scenario.

- Imagine that your Board has joined hands with other Boards and formed **The Grand Alliance for Compassion.**

- Reflect on the incredible power and influence such a coalition would possess. Imagine the change you can make, if you wanted to address the malaise and the angst that has gripped health care.

- You may rightly think it is unrealistic that such a grand alliance can be forged. But the American people rest their hope in each of you and in your individual Boards; as leaders, we ask for your assurance that you fully embrace person centered-care and will do your part to bring compassion back into health care.

- Many pioneers have successfully reintroduced humanity, magnanimity and benevolence; they have proved leaders matter in health care; their commitment and passion can move mountains and make way for compassion. However, without your active collaboration, these lone pioneers seem like pygmies battling Goliath.

- Consider the 691,400 physicians, 3.1 million nurses, nearly 5 million aides and countless number who work in health care. They have witnessed that their profession has let down consumers; they now see it abandoning its own as well. They know that a leader's commitment to compassion begins with the care and concern the leader shows for the care-giver. They see you as the last bastion of humanity and humane values in health care.

Your meditation may suggest to you several strategies to advance the cause of compassion. We request that within a month after the completion of the individual examinations of conscience, your Board makes a two-part public pledge. First, an affirmation that you fully re-commit yourself to restore humanity to health care; second, a proof of earnestness and sincerity that within the six months following you will launch an open and credible initiative to significantly advance the cause of compassion.

Projects, programs and events that help promote a culture of compassion are legion. And countless are the trails that lead you to that ideal. We have, with pride and joy, described or referenced many in this book.

Instead of reciting that glorious litany, we will list select actions you may duplicate, modify or draw inspiration from.

1. Re-visit your Board's mission statement. Consider centering it on compassionate care.

2. Amend the qualifications your Board requires in selecting, screening and installing new Board members. Require a prospective recruit to have a reputation, history or evidence of commitment to compassion.

3. Conduct an organizational audit to ensure that all policies, priorities, practices and protocols—every element from the mission statement to the job description of the maintenance worker—are in accord with the organization's mission and directed towards attaining it.

4. Sponsor research to develop user-friendly, concise measures of compassion, both quantitative and qualitative. These objective measures could be used for recruiting, training, evaluating, promoting and rewarding compassionate behavior of managers and staff within your Board or in affiliate organizations.

5. Make board meetings, agendas, budgets, priorities and policies, a practical enactment of your moral commitment to compassion. Leaders walk their talk. Encourage such consistency in your affiliate organizations.

6. Enrich the organizational culture—your Board's and your affiliates' organization's—with virtues related to compas-

sion: equality, fairness, empathy, open communication, politeness, courtesy, respect, trust and sharing.

7. Set up ways to counter and to deal firmly with conduct based on class, rank, race and privilege—the perpetual hurdles to compassion.

8. Celebrate, recognize, reward and propagate exceptional cases of benevolence, service, generosity and altruism. Conduct an annual audit of programs and initiatives to track the progress towards set goals pointing towards compassion.

9. Meet the human needs of the staff. Create an environment that is safe; respects each as an individual; encourages friendship among staff and with residents and families; publicly recognizes and rewards creativity and initiative; assists them rise to their potential, gives opportunity to grow as persons and professionals. Empower and delegate; cultivate openness and sharing matters of budget and policy. Include staff from every level in all important committees.

10. Aim at reaching the ideal of a fully person-centered care model. Give patients/residents full access to personal records, care plans and clinical notes. Make available complementary and alternative modes of healing. Let alternative healers give bed side care. Provide opportunity and a place for prayer, quiet and meditation. View families as clients needing help, take them as partners in care planning, care decisions, and care-giving. Encourage visitation at all hours and to bring home cooked meals.

A genuine pledge stands the test of sincerity. We appeal to the highest authorities in health care to sympathize with those within health care and with those without, who feel let down by those in whom we entrusted our health and well-being. We plead with them, well positioned and equipped as they are, to re-assure us by word and action that our trust has not been misplaced.

We look to them not to let the wounded Titanic sink further into the dark, lifeless morass, but to give it a decisive initial push and to set it on its return to the port of compassion.

George Burns once said, "Sincerity. If you can fake it, you've got it made!" By George! Not in health care!

Parkinson's Disease: My Nemesis, My Teacher

V. Tellis-Nayak

This narrative was published as a four-part series in the *Provider*. The editor's note that introduced the articles said, "We thought this compelling and poignant piece from Vivian Tellis-Nayak, PhD, was worth every drop of ink. This is the first installment of a new guest post about Tellis-Nayak's very personal struggle with Parkinson's disease [PD]. It will also be posted on *ProviderNation* on Nov. 4, 2013."

Part 1. November 2013

When PD gate-crashed into my life, it did not waste time. Its devastation started on day one. Its goal was total surrender, and its strategy was rapid fire.

Before I even thought of seeking medical help, PD had turned my world upside down.

I was unnerved seeing my familiar world standing wrong side up. Weak-kneed and adrift in an unfriendly terrain, I slipped, staggered, and stumbled trying to meet my professional obligations that I had handled effortlessly just yesterday.

My professor-student bond, among the most satisfying rewards for a teacher, began to congeal. Peer collegiality began to wilt and, with it, the camaraderie and mental high jinks I took delight in.

My ties within the family and with friends outside were stretched and strained.

PD turned my clock back. Mocking at my aspirations to be the kindly grandfather on the block, PD made me an infant and told me to start all over. I was to make sense of a world in shambles around me; I had to nurse my beaten ego. I had to salvage my self-image. All in all, an impossible mandate, enough to crush you into surrender and to make you slide into depression.

And that is what happened.

Melancholia's Drumbeat

PD snares sixty thousand new U.S. victims each year and drags nearly half of them into depression. The learned ones tell us that PD depression is more likely to occur with an early onset age, with greater left brain involvement, and lower cerebrospinal fluid levels of 5-hydroxyindoleacetic acid; it precipitates greater anxiety and lower-level self-punitive ideation.

Simply put, you go nuts when the chemical in your brain dries up and can no longer control the reward and pleasure centers.

I was relatively young and oblivious when PD sneaked in and began to play the reward-pleasure buttons in my left brain. I have lived by the dictum that biology is not destiny; I have bemoaned in written and spoken word that modern medicine too often discounts the human spirit and its power to transcend the frailties and limits of our body.

The pill, therefore, tasted more bitter when I learned that PD had broken through my spiritual barricades and had made me subservient to my errant body chemistry.

PD had me prostrate, despondent, and melancholic. I felt numb, dull, and hopeless, unable to savor the joy of life. I withdrew into my shell, not wanting to venture out into an unkind world. When I went out, I felt eyes were turned in my direction. I thought I heard people talking, *sotto voce*, about my condition.

My wife and I had for long anticipated our son's graduation from Northwestern as a jazz pianist. That celebratory day, however, I woke up insecure and timorous, emotionally out of synch with my family and unconnected with friends who had come from faraway places to partake in the joys of the occasion. I tried my best, and all I could muster was weak, clammy handshakes and squeaky "Hellos."

None of us—family, friends, or I—had any inkling that PD was at the joysticks again, gleefully tinkering with my life.

Melancholia stalked me through sleepless nights and joyless days. It kept up a relentless drumbeat: you cannot be you again; you cannot be healed.

Although demoralized and diffident, I acceded to my wife and accompanied her to a professional conference to present a paper we had co-authored. I stood in front of the attending scholars, feeling vulnerable, with a vapid look, and drained of the last drop of the confidence of the seasoned author I displayed on such occasions.

I survived the ordeal only because at every punctuation mark, I looked up and felt reassured by the subtle nods from my wife seated in the front row.

PD: An Acid Test

PD is at its vilest when it comes to personal relations. Very early, PD targets your strongest bastion of hope and support. It strains the marital bond and warps familial ties. PD, in fact, is an acid test of the resilience of family cohesion.

PD's devilry sows mistrust and doubt; it rasps and grates on the family bond until it is raw and stretches it to its breaking point.

That sets up a depth charge, which results in new fissures that widen dormant family fault lines. Scars from long-forgotten intemperate words, resentments, and petty jealousies now fester again and prove fatal to all but the most robust relationships.

How many marriages, joyous unions, and liaisons have succumbed to the savagery of PD? I dare not contemplate.

I survived PD's gauntlet of depression. My wife and I discovered that our mutual devotion had steel and stamina that we had not suspected. Although buffeted and bruised, our commitment triumphed over PD's guile and sagacity.

We had sailed troubled waters before. Our two odd biographies racing on different trajectories had converged in a mixed ethnic marriage despite harsh reaction and punitive threats.

From that inauspicious starting line, our life together had been a sprint down an obstacle course. We have lived through social rejection, cultural contradictions, serious health challenges, and the frustrations of fostering seventeen children. None of these ordeals matched the fury and ferocity that PD directed toward us.

I count my blessings. The most precious of them is my partner in life, Mary, impossibly gregarious in nature, eternally sunny in disposition, and with a bit of an inflated can-do approach to life.

It is a favor from the gods that she is a geriatric nurse, and it is a sign of their fondness for me that she is quite a few years younger than me. She keeps me well fed on recipes she learned from my mother. She sees that I am attired and suited appropriately for the occasion. She fights off PD's new incursions like a provoked lioness.

Part 2. December 2013

Paradoxically, the more solid a marital bond, the higher the toll PD exacts. I have seen firsthand what it takes for a wife to care for an ailing husband. Her burden gets heavier as I depend on her more and more in matters of personal care. Mary plans, makes appointments, and drives me 108 miles to and fro for regular visits with my neurologist, a godsend, whom she selected after much research.

She buys and dispenses the six daily doses of twelve different meds. She fights pitched battles with insurance companies and Medicare. She has never missed a deadline for documentation.

Meanwhile, I gradually withdraw, by PD orders, from doing household chores, thereby increasing her share of it. And all this, mind you, while she pursues a professional career with heavy travel demands.

The Breaking Point

There are times when you catch a glimpse of her as overwhelmed, irritated, and chafing under her cross that weighs heavier each day. Two weeks ago, I watched her inching to the edge. She was out early, running errands; she returned with a heavy load of groceries. Not letting me exert, she put away the groceries without help.

The next hour we were speeding down U.S. 90, Mary at the wheel and grandkids in tow, for an obligatory get-together with the in-laws living three hours away in Indiana.

When you are at the ripe end of your sixties, you do not brim over with youthful stamina. So by day's end, Mary was tense and her dander up. She clenched her fist and, with righteous anger, cursed PD. "Damn you!" she said hotly. "Why have you laid this cross on me?" Then she turned toward me and with unfocussed resentment said, "I am ready to break. I admire your courage. But I am sinking." Then she cried. A bit later, she apologized.

Being philosophically inclined, I sought a rational answer. Why, I puzzled, has nature endowed wives and mothers with only two, not four, hands?

I have never seen it, but friends have confirmed my suspicion: PD has brought Mary to tears, shed privately and in silence as she sees me slide in health, speech, and function.

On occasion, when she is certain I won't take hurt, she lets me peek into her soul, ruffled by the anticipation of what PD holds in store for her: a longer life without her soul mate of forty-three years (and counting), without the partner who took delight in her success, and without the handyman who took on every problem in the house with a bravado that exceeded his skill.

I am blessed, indeed, that she cares for me exquisitely, even to a fault. But I too grieve in silence that the gods gave her youth but only at the price of being a caregiver half her married life and a longer, lonely widowhood.

I am put off at God, as I am with Mother Nature. Why do so many long-suffering, deserving wives and mothers never attain canonical sainthood?

Angels and Mother Superior

PD has brought me other insights and revelations. Receiving good care from your spouse, I have rightly concluded, is not entirely an unmixed blessing, especially if your consort is well-schooled, smart, Irish, and an ex-nun. A hired caregiver, like Kathleen, who has helped us out, would take it in stride and humor my quirks and peccadilloes, if I had any.

Not unlike my guardian angel, Kathleen coaxes me to stick to my regimen, but she understands when I don't. When she is on duty, I take shortcuts, I (metaphorically) let my hair down (I am as bald as a new-laid egg), and I flirt with minor temptations that add fun to life, especially when you give in to them.

When K, the angel, goes off duty, Mother Superior Mary comes aboard, ruler in hand. Instantly, the script changes, and I assume a role akin to Mary's little lamb.

Through the thick and thin of family life, Mary has learned all there is about me. She knows my minor vices, and she has steered me away from the seven capital sins.

She is well versed in the clever games spouses play in marital power tugs. So I weigh the odds when I want her help. Every time I call out for help, a handy app in her mind instantly analyzes the tenor, tone, and tempo of my petition and determines if my plea was a moan of self-pity, a ruse to get attention, or a genuine plea for help.

The next second she is by my side with a response suited for the occasion—lending me a caring and helping hand or admonishing me on a familiar theme: how "growing old is not the same as growing up."

Treasure of Human Life

In ways both symbolic and real, the rhythm of family life adjusts to the demands PD makes. Our son has not found how to cope with the way his dad has declined so quickly and visibly in function and gait. Our two grandkids have never seen their grandpa in his pre-PD glory. They wonder how I can talk incoherently as a toddler, demand as much attention as does a baby, and still receive the care and respect due to a family antique. Grandma gets more than her share of hugs and smudgy kisses as I wait for the leftovers. To the kids, Grandma is fantasy come true—Fairy Godmother and Mrs. Santa Claus wrapped in one—while Grandpapa serves as the clandestine source of candy, the forbidden fruit banned by overcautious, thoroughly mistaken parents.

As PD has ordained, I am no longer the wise Solomon who set the direction for the family and had the final word. Now, my kind family spares me the exertion of planning family events, vacations, and travel. Still, it stings when they forget to tell me their decision and I learn of it from the neighbor.

I have to face it, even in the family, I have fallen in status, although not from grace. When preparing for a road trip or for a picnic, Mary anticipates the needs of each. She packs three bags, one for the grandkids, one for our four-pound pooch, and one for me.

In sum, PD has not let up and is still hell-bent on bringing me to my knees. In ways vile and vicious, it has attempted to crumple my professional life and to crush my personal world.

It has knocked me off pedestals and has brought tears, pain, and sorrow to those dearest to me.

This meanest of teachers has made me walk through the dark tunnel of depression and the valley of defeat and shame. This searing internship, however, has taught me to cherish the gift of human life—the indomitable human spirit that can lift you from the ashes, the power of love that can rescue you from misery, and the healing bonds of family and friends—angels that can make you whole again.

Part 3. January 2014

Parkinson's disease (PD) has dragged me through hellfire; it has wrecked my body and tested my soul. This ordeal has taught me much about life in general and about matters both great and trivial. Following are some highlights of my life with PD and of what this mean teacher taught me about modern medicine, its marvels and pitfalls.

It happened ten days before Christmas 2009. I was somewhere over the rainbow, in deep slumber, when I felt a hand pressing my shoulder and heard a voice, "Dr. Tellis-Nayak! I want you to be awake!"

Reality dawned ray by ray—I couldn't budge; I was belted down, my skull was in a vise inside a steel trap bolted down to the metal bed. Around me stood six men and women, all oozing smarts. I saw, on my left, a compact figure wearing a white gown and a triumphant smile. "How do you feel?" Dr. V asked. Suddenly, reality crashed in, and everything came into focus.

I was at the hospital getting a brain tune-up from Dr. V. I was under conscious sedation and told to stay awake, but trusting my brain in Dr. V's hands, I had slid into a midday siesta on my personal Fantasy Island.

PD had sneaked up on me; my left-hand tremors started in 1995. PD turned my world upside down, and it directed its unmitigated fury toward my professional life; it took aim at areas where I felt particularly proud and would hurt the most.

Worse, PD made me watch in slow motion my descent into a personal hell. The professor, the researcher, and the public speaker in me suffered exquisite mortification. My strut gone, now I shuffled my way to the podium; I stood there unstable and ungainly, my left hand shaking against my will, my voice barely louder than a squeak, my speech reduced to a mumble, my words slurring; I could not read my scrawl on the blackboard.

My medical regimen had blunted PD's attack but did not halt its advance. My intellectual and spiritual defenses did not match its resolve to drag me toward the black hole of helplessness, meaning-lessness, self-pity, and despair.

On the verge of surrender, I reached out to Dr. V for a brain tune-up. He recommended DBS (deep brain stimulation). I signed on immediately.

Resetting Brain Circuits

DBS is based on the evidence that each human action (motor, mem-ory, or cognition) is modulated by a specific brain circuit located in a specific brain area. DBS works as a radio works. You turn one dial to locate the station and another to turn the volume up or down. Similarly, you locate the brain area whose circuit is linked to a spe-cific human activity. You implant a pace setter to stabilize, accelerate, or slow that circuit and so to regulate the activity associated with it.

Two professors at Grenoble, France, introduced DBS to the world in 1987 as an effective treatment for PD. It is now used to treat other movement disorders and neurological and psychiatric condi-tions. About one hundred thousand DBS implants have been done worldwide.

I was at the hospital the night before my early morning date with DBS. Dr. V planned the event to unfold in two steps. First, they wrapped a metal trap around my skull, calling it a halo.

The halo bolted down my head immovably as the medical cognoscenti mapped my brain; the coordinates set and traced the optimal route to my sub thalamic region. They numbed my scalp, cut a five-inch gash, and with a press-drill a bit fancier than my True Value version, they bore a hole the size of a quarter into my skull.

Human brains have no pain feelers. So under conscious sedation, I was supposed to stay awake and enjoy the sight and sounds of my own demolition. I chose to snore away in dreamland.

High Drama

The next part was high drama. The docs held an electrode (metal rod) at the hole in my head (front-right and due north from the eye), angled it about forty-five degrees, and drove it through the center of the brain toward a pea-sized target in the subthalamus basement of the brain.

The mindless invader decimated my brain cells in its path and sent them into oblivion, each emitting a digital dying wail. I mourned the IQ points I lost in operation DBS.

With the rod lodged close to its destination, Dr. V pulled me back from my dreamy escape. His smiley-like smile told me the train had arrived, and now he needed my help to pick the right platform where it should be stationed.

For the next fifteen minutes, he twisted and turned my left hand in every direction, while Dr. O, his partner in this invasion, jabbed, stabbed, and poked around my brain till they found the optimal spot to park the hot rod.

To spare me the gruesome sight of the last scene, the medicine men tripped my main fuse and blanked me out. They cut open a pouch below my right collar bone, nested in it a thick credit-card-sized battery with a trailing cable, which they buried under the skin along a path from my chest, winding up behind the ear, and joining it to the electrode under the skull.

My traumatized brain protested, swelled, and delayed the turning on of the switch buried in my chest. They gave me a remote control that turned the stimulator in my brain on or off.

I take care to keep it out of reach of my grandkids, lest they should get ideas and use it as a joystick.

Belles and Cherubs

The gurney brought me to the recovery room looking like Lazarus swaddled in bandages, staggering out of the sepulcher.

I was relieved that I survived the eight-hour storming of my defenseless brain and was buoyed by the company of Mary, my long-suffering personal nurse and bride of over four decades.

Back in my room, a bevy of belles—bright-faced, freshly minted young nurses—greeted the return of their most compliant patient, who, since last evening, had let them poke needles into me; draw blood from me; and thrust thermometers, meds, and other foreign objects into my orifices.

I felt blessed among these women.

My son had dropped in the night before and had fortified my soul for the ordeal. This evening, he came with his consort and their two bouncy cherubs in tow. The next two hours were pure chaos—laughter, son, and horse play as the cherubs revived Grandpa Lazarus.

Jocelyn, RN, had recorded my runaway blood pressure a little before the kids came. She dropped by to track it again as they were about to depart. Her jaw dropped to the floor: my blood pressure had plummeted down to normal!

Do kids have a role to play in brain surgery? Why do hospital visiting rules for kids vary so widely? Some hospitals encourage families to visit, when some others cannot seem to bear the sight of them.

I wondered which of these policies and practices were rooted in firm evidence and which in common sense.

Part 4. February 2014

My introduction to DBS also introduced me to a wide difference among hospital policies and safety protocols. In a tertiary care hospital, the sanctuary of modern medicine, I witnessed homage being paid to the false gods of irrationality.

I was at the center of a scary incongruity, only hours before surgery. I was at the hospital late Wednesday evening, sporting a confident smile that masked my diffident heart. To combat PD, the docs were to plant a sentinel inside my skull, and I had no clue how my brain would accept its new roommate.

On the Edge of Fiasco

I perked up when they brought in, as a compromise, not the bed we requested but a reclining chair so my wife, Mary, could be with me on the presurgery night. A parade of clinicians drifted in and out. They checked my vitals, told us what I could eat and drink (a strict fast beginning at midnight), and what meds to take (strictly no PD drugs until after surgery—they seriously hinder the optimal positioning of the deep brain device).

The parade continued through the night; new faces materialized by my bed at unpredictable intervals. Each time they nudged me awake, introduced themselves, and checked my vitals for the hundredth time.

Mary, a reputed expert in person-centered care, was aghast; none of the well-meaning clinicians were aware that they were complying with a misguided protocol that disrupted her husband's rest on the night before major surgery.

Her conclusion: "This system is thoughtless and ill planned. Could it be they have not heard of patient-centeredness and of customer service?"

It's 5:00 a.m. I am up again, this time fully awake to be prepped for surgery.

At the tail end of the parade, friendly Nicole, RN, shows up, chitchats, and graciously asks, "Are you ready for your first dose of medicine?"

Ever vigilant, Mary is up instantly, sitting bolt upright. The nurse in her wants to know: "And what medicine is that?" Nicole reads out, word after deliberate word, the prescription. In effect, she detonates a bomb: "It is his first dose of Parkinson's drugs."

The verbal cat fight that followed was great theatrics, but it should not have been a part of my preop prep. Mary puts her foot down and will not let me take the medicine, and Nicole invokes the protocol that includes no hold on the presurgical administration of the medicine. An accord is reached, and Mary is declared the hero. She had forestalled a disaster. An expensive eight-hour surgical event presided over by the high priests of medicine, backed up by state-of-the-art support system—all this would have come to naught and would have triggered a cascade of financial, legal, and ethical consequences.

Mary had spared me the clinical fallout from a tragic medical fiasco.

Weak Links and Pitfalls

It unnerved me to see up close how one weak link can unfasten a fine-tuned intricate procedure. My spirits sank further when I discovered there might be other kinks in the system.

All system are go. I am at ground zero, waiting for a stranger I have never met to come and drill a hole in my head.

The surgeon arrives on time. He coasts in with an unexpectedly jolly demeanor; he greets the assembled acolytes and cheerfully lobs a question somewhere in my direction, "So which side do I drill today?"

The casual question hit me like a ton of bricks. "Which side? He doesn't know?" An inaudible scream welled from my depths, and my mind conjured up an image of a scalper who does his routine on one nameless head and moves to the next.

His question probably was part of a best practice among clinicians to avoid identity errors. Still, his demeanor, words, and tone did little to reassure the befuddled and unnerved patient at his mercy.

A credentialed brain surgeon who flouts elementary rules of psychology and courtesy—how does a hospital monitor such behavior and measure its effects?

Earlier that morning I watched in living color another misalignment: a technical compliance to protocol out of synch with the needs of the patient and of the moment.

On the way to surgery, my gurney made stops; nurses, interns, and other unknowns took their turn with me. They asked me questions. Again and again I told them my name and date of birth, wondering why, at this stage, they were not convinced that I was really me. I took note. Most questioners showed concern but were not focused. For sure, they were not hanging on to my answers.

They kept asking their scripted questions. I mumbled inaudible or incorrect answers. A lower-rung functionary sensed my playfulness and winked me his approval. None of the others caught on; they had followed protocol, and that was that.

I witnessed other incongruous encounters at every turn.

When medics meet patients and their families in a hospital setting, they are usually not aware that their demeanor, even a single word or gesture, may have an unintended blighting effect.

The anxious and sometimes traumatized patient looks for a meaning in every nod, shrug, or smile. A casual observation, a hint of impatience, interrupting the patient's narrative—the silent vocabulary of our everyday body language—may carry a dire message or may seem to trivialize the patient's concern.

High-tech medicine should not be incompatible with the caring touch.

My surgery complete, I ran smack into yet another glitch. A considerate, muscled orderly wheeled me to the recovery room. Mary was waiting for me, looking her happiest; the doc had told her the surgery was an A-plus success. The orderly aligned the gurney with the recovery room bed. He gingerly stepped aside and politely asked me to scoot over from the gurney to the bed.

Instantly Mary's spine went ramrod straight—her Irish was up. "What are you saying?" she demanded. "My husband has just had brain surgery. He cannot transfer to the bed by himself!"

The orderly visibly shrank. Timidly he whispered, "Nobody told me that!"

Untapped Resources

Back to home life, the surprises continued. The hospital that offered me a course (call it high-tech success and low-tech failure) on the promise and perils of modern medicine makes the honors list of the top safest hospitals in the country.

A national magazine hails the technical and behavioral innovations in these hospitals to combat hospital-based infection and human error that harm one in three patients and kill 180,000 every year.

Sadly, I find it does not refer to a single hospital that has partnered with staff, patients, and families and has viewed safety from their unique vantage point.

The glitches I encountered all occurred below the radar of the hospital's state-of-the-art, risk-alert system.

My DBS surgery, by any standard, was a modern medical miracle. That feat was accomplished despite the pitfalls that lurked around every corner—that was no less a miracle.

Medical Milestones: The Past 500 Years

Founding & Major Figures	Birth–Death Years	Discoveries
1. Elucidation of Human Anatomy and Physiology		
William Harvey	1578–1657	Blood circulation
Alfred Blalock	1899–1964	Advanced open heart surgery
André Cournand	1895–1988	Clinical catheterization
Andreas Vesalius	1514–1564	Anatomical treatise
Charles Hufnagel	1916–1989	Advanced open heart surgery
Elliott Cutler	1888–1947	Advanced open heart surgery
Robert Gross	1905–1988	Advanced open heart surgery
Stephen Hales	1677–1761	Measured blood pressure in a horse
Werner Forssmann	1904–1979	Heart catheterization
2. Discovery of Cells and Substructures		
Ernst Ruska	1906–1988	Electron microscope
Rudolf Virchow	1821–1902	Advanced cell biology
Antonie van Leeuwenhoek	1632–1723	Saw animacules (bacteria)
Carl von Rokitansky	1804–1878	Cell biology and disease process
George Palade	1912–2008	Subcellular elements like mitochondria
Ludwig Aschoff	1866–1942	Cell biology, disease processes
Matthias Schleiden	1804–1881	Described animal cells
Robert Hooke	1635–1703	Plant cells
Theodor Schwann	1810–1882	Animal cells
3. Elucidation of the Chemistry of Life		
Thomas Willis	1621–1675	"Every disease has some ferment"
Amadeo Avogadro	1776–1856	Avogadro's law of atomic weights
Antoine Lavoisier	1743–1794	Laid ground for germ theory
Hans Krebs	1900–1981	Discovered the citric acid cycle
Jöns Jacob Berzelius	1779–1848	Advanced germ theory

MEDICAL MILESTONES: THE PAST 500 YEARS

Leonor Michaelis	1875–1949	Expressed enzyme reactions mathematically
Maud Menten	1879–1960	Expressed enzyme reactions mathematically
Otto Warburg	1883–1970	Pathways of metabolism

4. Application of Statistics to Medicine

Blaise Pascal	1623–1662	Probability theory used in epidemiology
Pierre de Fermat	1607–1665	Probability theory used in epidemiology
James Lind	1716–1794	Effectively treated scurvy
Jerzy Neyman	1894–1981	Theories of estimation and testing
John Graunt	1620–1674	Concept of inference from a sample
John Snow	1813–1858	Applied statistics to fight cholera
Carl Friedrich Gauss	1777–1855	Statistical reasoning
Sir Richard Doll	1912–2005	Pioneered study of physicians' smoking
Sir Ronald Fisher	1890–1962	Randomization to avoid bias
Thomas Bayes	1701–1761	Probability in inductive reasoning

5. Development of Anesthesia

Harold Griffith	1894–1985	Used muscle relaxants during surgery
Horace Wells	1815–1848	Nitrous oxide used as anesthesia
Sir James Young Simpson	1811–1870	Administered chloroform to woman in childbirth
William T. G. Morton	1819–1868	First to use ether as anesthesia

6. Discovery of Microbe Disease Link

Louis Pasteur	1822–1895	Made bacteriology a science
Robert Koch	1843–1910	Isolated agents of cholera and TB; authored "Koch's postulates"
Joseph Lister	1827–1912	Carbolic acid as antiseptic during surgery

7. Elucidation of Inheritance, Genetics

Gregor Mendel	1822–1884	Segregated traits in peas
Sir Archibald Garrod	1857–1936	Inborn errors of metabolism are inherited
Boris Ephrussi	1901–1979	Genes specify enzymes
Colin MacLeod	1909–1972	Found that DNA is the genetic material

David Baltimore	b. 1938	Reverse transcriptase: converts RNA into DNA
Dickinson Richards	1895–1973	Clinical catheterization
Edward Tatum	1909–1975	Genes specify enzymes
Erwin Chargaff	1905–2002	Bases of DNA and rules of base pairing
Francis Crick	1916–2004	Double helix
Francois Jacob	1920–2013	DNA to RNA
Frederick Sanger	1918–2013	Decoded sequence of bases in DNA
George Beadle	1903–1989	Showed genes specify enzymes
Howard Temin	1934–1994	Reverse transcriptase: converts RNA into DNA
Jacques Monod	1910–1976	DNA to protein via messenger RNA
James Watson	b. 1928	Double helix
Linus Pauling	1901–1994	Sickle cell mutation
Maclyn McCarty	1911–2005	Found that DNA is the genetic material
Maurice Wilkins	1916–2004	Double helix
Rosalind Franklin	1920–1958	X-ray diffraction led to discovery of the double helix
Oswald Avery	1877–1955	Found that DNA is the genetic material
Thomas Hunt Morgan	1866–1945	Drew maps of genes along chromosomes
Walter Gilbert	b. 1932	Decoding DNA sequence
8. Knowledge of the Immune System		
Emil von Behring	1854–1917	Developed a diphtheria antitoxin and discovered antibodies
Albert Sabin	1906–1993	Made live-weakened polio vaccine
Élie Metchnikoff	1845–1916	Identified phagocytes, offered cellular theory of immunity
Frederick Robbins	1916–2003	Isolated polio virus to pave way for vaccine
John Enders	1897–1985	Made measles vaccine
Jonas Salk	1914–1995	Made killed-virus vaccine
Kitasato Shibasaburo	1853–1931	Diphtheria antitoxin serum
Michael Heidelberger	1888–1991	Laid foundation for pneumococcal vaccines
Thomas Weller	1915–2008	Cultivated poliomyelitis virus in a test tube

9. Development of Body Imaging		
Wilhelm Konrad Röentgen	1845–1923	X-rays, won first Nobel prize for physics in 1901
Stage 1		Imaging techniques to define the anatomic features and functions of the internal organs
Stage 2		Angiography delineates the interior of the heart and blood vessels
Stage 3		Imaging directly guides cancer therapy and minimally invasive surgery
10. Discovery of Antimicrobial Agents		
Paul Ehrlich	1854–1915	Salvarsan to treat syphilis; showed dyes are antimicrobial
Sir Alexander Fleming	1881–1955	Staph bacteria inhibited by a mold, penicillium
Sir Ernst Chain	1906–1979	Purified penicillin for human use
Gerhard Domagk	1895–1964	Red dye prontosil cures strep infections; led to sulfa drugs
Howard Florey	1898–1968	Purified penicillin for clinical use
René Dubos	1901–1982	Antibiotic in an organism in the soil
Selman Waksman	1888–1973	Found streptomycin in soil organisms
11. Development of Molecular Pharmacotherapy		
Paul Ehrlich	1854–1915	Coined terms "chemotherapy" and "magic bullet" from infections to cancer
Alfred Gilman	1908–1984	Found nitrogen mustard ("mustard gas") helped treat lymphomas
Barnett Rosenberg	1926–2009	Discovered the anticancer drug cisplatin
Charles Huggins	1901–1997	Showed value of orchiectomy for prostate cancer
Frederick S. Philips	1923–1984	Studied effects of gases to treat malignant tumors
Sir James Black	1924–2010	His work led to the development of beta blockers
Sidney Farber	1903–1973	Father of chemotherapy
Sir George Beatson	1848–1933	Used oophorectomy for breast cancer

The Business Case for Compassion in Health Care

Christian Mason, a decades-long friend, embodies an unerring entrepreneurial instinct guided by a compassionate heart. No surprise that right in the middle of pursuing a doctorate, he launches a highly successful program that promotes altruism in the community. We asked Chris to make a business case for compassion in health care. He wrote the following,

V. Tellis-Nayak
Mary Tellis-Nayak

The Business Case for Compassion in Health Care

By Christian A. Mason
Chair, National Center for Assisted Living/
American Health Care Association

How do we meet the challenge of enhancing patient experience while reducing the per capita cost of health care? The answer is by reigniting the flame of compassion in health care. To accomplish this, we must make the business case for why compassion must be at the center of any health care debate.

Take for example Barry, a functional quadriplegic living in a nursing center in Alabama. When first introduced to Barry, I was a new and inexperienced administrator who didn't understand the boundaries of the job. Barry had been a college football player before his accident and had loved outdoor activities such as camping and fishing. When Barry asked me why he could not still do those things I was at a loss to give him any answer other than why not? Putting compassion first became the impetus behind the development of a resident camping program that culminated in taking an entire nursing community camping. The impact on residents, staff, and family was significant. It also turned out to be significant to the bottom line. This community became known for compassion and as such was the preferred choice for care in the city.

As human beings, we expect care and compassion to be cornerstones of our health care experiences. Mencius says, "No man is devoid of a heart sensitive to the sufferings of others… whoever is devoid of the heart of compassion is not human." Compassion is often viewed as the deep feeling of connectedness with the experience of human suffering we see firsthand from serving patients and residents each and every day. This personal knowledge evokes a moral response in us to bring comfort to the sufferer. It is this ethical perspective of sympathy and compassion that health care workers bring to their place of work daily.

Moral psychology emphasizes the human side of the business. These include how personal feelings affect and are influenced by organizational culture and human motivation. This can be seen by how we relate to other human beings when they are most vulnerable. So what happens when this is stifled or downplayed within health care organizations or a personal health care experience? In both cases, a void is created. The patient equates this with a subpar health care experience. This is often translated into negative satisfaction and shows up in a lack of repeat business. They view the health care provider or system as uncaring. Likewise, when compassion is not viewed as a critical organizational priority, employees show negative satisfaction towards the organization. Ethically, the organization is viewed as cold, sterile or worse. Health care organizations must understand the intimate link between compassion, sympathy, understanding, and the sense of belonging that comes from a community of people caring for each other. When organizations fail to accomplish this, employees often see the organization as putting profits before people. Taking such a view is both shortsighted and lacking in understanding of how compassion can fuel an organization to success.

In Tacoma, Washington a new program was recently launched named Wellness Made Easy. The purpose of the program is to promote wellness, provide primary health care services to residents and their families, staff and their families, and neighbors from the surrounding area, and to engage individuals in a dialogue centered on helping others. A central theme of the program is people helping people. Members are rewarded for helping others and spreading compassion through volunteer efforts. Rewards include such things as no deductibles or copays in the clinic, recognition, and access to deeply discounted programs, products, and services. In the first week of operations, over 500 individuals signed up to participate. Showing compassion is also good business. The success of this program could add as much as 50 percent to the valuation of the property over time.

To understand the value of compassion in the workplace we need only look at history. Adam Smith, generally considered one of the most influential business philosophers, speaks of "moral sentiment" as essential for business and "sympathy" as a critical virtue. Aristotle viewed sympathy and compassion as nobler feelings inherent in humanity. While it is in the interest of leaders and organizations to act in a compassionate manner for image and ethical reasons, it is also important they do so for financial reasons. Rational thought and sound business strategy should support organizations focus on care and compassion rather than demoting it to a footnote in the company's business plan. Compassion is not a commodity to be doled out only to those who can afford it. Health care leaders must ask the question: Is the patient being forgotten? Successful health care organizations have returned their focus to the four founding pillars of compassion, solidarity, equity and social justice. Moral leaders must respond with their heads as well as their hearts.

Employees nurtured in a compassionate organizational culture develop an authentic sense of community; that is, they relate to each other as members of a group that is committed to positive ideals and actions, and they exhibit a real empathy for each other. Take for example Pam, a charge nurse working the evening shift in a care community. Pam was a single mom trying to raise two children on her own. Her dream was to own her own home. Yet no matter how much she saved she never had quite enough. That is until the idea of using vacation, sick, and paid time off as a savings account was introduced. By permitting employees to save and accumulate time rather than use it or lose it Pam was able to put away enough for her down payment. So it was no wonder that when the community needed help to care for residents when flooding occurred during a hurricane that Pam was the first one to arrive and the last one to leave.

This simple gesture of compassion translated into a strong workforce where low turnover, high levels of satisfaction, and strong ties to patient engagement could often be found. Let us not forget that it takes tremendous courage to serve those in need. Employees must not only keep their hearts open, but those hearts must be big enough to hold the suffering of others. This means having passion for our work, compassion for the people we serve, empathy for the people with whom we work, and the courage to do it day in and day out over and over again. Don't our employees deserve the same?

To summarize the business case for compassion one need only remind oneself of the story of the Good Samaritan. The story teaches us the values of solidarity, equity, compassion and social justice. It also highlights the difference between the mission and business of health care. While the business of health care focuses on clinical precision, innovation, teamwork, and accountability, the mission focuses on equity, respect, collaboration, patient centeredness, and compassion. The mission is the driving force behind the business. It contains the values that guide all caregivers: compassion, empathy, community, solidarity, and social justice. While health care organizations periodically confuse the concepts of business and mission, it is mission that drives success.

Endnotes

0.01   The Osler Symposia, "Sir William Osler & His Inspirational Words" (Web page, accessed June 13, 2016, www.oslersymposia.org/about-Sir-William-Osler.html.

1.01   Pinecrest Medical Care Facility, N-15995 Main Street, Powers, MI, 49874 (www.pinecrestmcf.org).

1.02   It's Never 2 Late, 7330 S Alton Way, Englewood, CO 80112 (www. in2l.com).

1.03   St. Joseph's Home, 80 West Northwest Highway, Palatine, IL 6006 (www.littlesistersofthepoorpalatine.org).

1.04   Planetree, 130 Division St., Derby, CT 06418 (www.planetree.org).

2.01   Max Weber, "The Ideal Type," School of Social Sciences, Cardiff University (Web page, accessed February 22, 2016), www.cf.ac.uk/socsi/undergraduate/introsoc/weber7.html.

2.02   W. Andrews (graphic), "The high cost of medical procedures in the U.S.," The Washington Post (data sourced from International Federation of Health Plans), March 2, 2012, www.washingtonpost.com/business/2012/03/01/gIQAvuEdmR_graphic.html.

2.03   Debt.org, "Hospital and Surgery Costs" (Web page, accessed February 22, 2016), www.debt.org/medical/hospital-surgery-costs/.

2.04 Jason Kane, "Health Costs: How the U.S. Compares With Other Countries," PBS, October 22, 2012.

3.01 J. B. Mckinlay and L. D. Marceau, "The End of the Golden Age of Doctoring," *International Journal of Health Services*, 2002, 32(2): 379–416.

3.02 D. M. Jolliffe, "A History of the Use of Arsenicals in Man," *Journal of the Royal Society of Medicine*, 1993, 86(5): 287–289.

3.03 J. A. Hayman, "Diagnosis: Darwin's Illness Revisited," *British Medical Journal*, December 14, 2009, 339:b4968.

3.04 J. Marrcotty, "Lincoln's Medicine Contained 9000 Times More Mercury Than Safe," *Star Tribune*, July 18, 2001.

3.05 C. Lobel, "Sylvester Graham and Antebellum Diet Reform," The Gilder Lehrman Institute of American History, www.gilderlehrman.org/history-by-era/first-age-reform/essays/sylvester-graham-and-antebellum-diet-reform.

3.06 International Wellness Directory, "The History of Medicine 1800–1850," Minnesota Wellness Publications, 2013, www.mnwelldir.org/docs/history/history03.htm.

3.07 R. J. Tannenbaum, *Health and Wellness in Colonial America*, Greenwood, 2012.

3.08 A. J. Youngson, "Medical Education in the Later 19th Century: The Science Take-Over," *Medical Education*, November 1989, 23(6):480–91.

3.09 A. Flexner, *Medical Education in the United States and Canada: A Report to the Carnegie Foundation for the Advancement of Teaching*, 1910.

3.10 D. Hiatt and C. Stockton, "The Impact of the Flexner Report on the Fate of Medical Schools in North America After 1909," *Journal of American Physicians and Surgeons*, Summer 2003, 8(2): 37-40.

3.11 M. M. Wooster, "John Rockefeller Jr.," Philanthropy Roundtable, http://www.philanthropyroundtable.org/ almanac/hall_of_fame/john_d._rockefeller_jr; and J. S. Gordon, "John Rockefeller Sr.", Philanthropy Roundtable, http://www.philanthropyroundtable.org/ alm.

3.12 D. Ullman, *Discovering Homeopathy: Your Introduction to the Science and Art of Homeopathic Medicine* (Second Revised Edition), North Atlantic Books, January 1, 1993.

3.13 References are available online; see for example, Robert Wood Johnson Foundation, "Poll Finds Majority of Americans View Their Health Care Positively, While Many Still Report Problems with Costs, Quality, and Access to Services," February 29, 2016, www.rwjf.org/ en/library/articles-and-news/2016/02/patient-percep-tions-vary-across-seven-states.html.

3.14 NPR, Robert Wood Johnson Foundation, and Harvard School of Public Health, Poll: "Sick in America" (Summary), May 2012.

3.15 National Center for Health Statistics, *National Health Interview Survey*, Centers for Disease Control and Prevention, 2007.

3.16 Centers for Disease Control and Prevention, "Morbidity and Mortality Weekly Report MMWR" (Web page), October 9, 2015, No. 39.

3.17 AARP and National Center for Complementary and Alternative Medicine, *Complementary and Alternative Medicine: What People Aged 50 And Older Discus with Their Health Care Providers* (Consumer Survey Report), U.S. Department of Health and Human Services and National Institutes of Health, April 2011.

3.18 The Physicians Foundation, *A Survey of America's Physicians: Practice Patterns and Perspectives* (survey conducted by Merritt Hawkins), September 2014; and H. Lu, A. E. While, and K. L. Barriball, "Job Satisfaction Among Nurses: A Literature Review," *International journal of Nursing Studies*, February 2005, 42(2): 211–223.

3.19 J. T. James, "A New, Evidence-Based Estimate of Patient Harms Associated with Hospital Care," *Journal of Patient Safety,* September 2013, 9(3).

3.20 I. Illich, "Chapter 1: The Epidemics of Modern Medicine," *Medical Nemesis: The Expropriation of Health,* Pantheon, August 12, 1982.

3.21 The Physicians Foundation, *A Survey of America's Physicians: Practice Patterns and Perspectives* (survey conducted by Merritt Hawkins), September 2014.

4.01 P. E. Ruskin, M.D., "Aging and Caring," *Journal of the American Medical Association*, October 22, 1997, 278(16):1384.

4.02 S. A. Levine and B. Lown, "'Armchair' Treatment of Acute Coronary Thrombosis," *Journal of the American Medical Association*, April 19, 1952, 148(16): 1365-1369.

4.03 Bio., "Florence Nightingale Biography (Nurse 1820–1910)," www.biography.com/people/florence-nightingale-9423539.

4.04 D. M. Berwick, M.D., M.P.P., *Escape Fire: Lessons for the Future of Health Care*, The Commonwealth Fund, 2002.

4.05 "Compassion Doesn't Cost a Dollar," *New Zealand Listene*r, April 11, 2009, pp. 20–21.

4.06 M. Kakutani, "Review: In 'Do No Harm,' A Brain Surgeon Tells All," *The New York Times*, May 18, 2015.

4.07 J. Aleccia, "Nurse's suicide highlights twin tragedies of medical errors," NBC News, Jun 27, 2011.

4.08 *Ibid.*

4.09 T. Brown, "When Nurses Make Mistakes," *The New York Times*, July 6, 2011.

4.10 V. Tellis-Nayak, "Who Will Care for the Caregivers?" *Health Progress,* November-December 2005, 866:37-43.

4.11 The Physicians Foundation, *A Survey of America's Physicians: Practice Patterns and Perspectives* (survey conducted by Merritt Hawkins), September 2014.

4.12 L. Barclay, M.D., "Medical Interns Spend Very Little Time at Patient Bedsides," *Medscape Medical News*, April 25, 2013.

4.13 A. Kelly, J. Conell-Price, K. Covinsky, I. StijacicCenzer, A. Chang, W. J. Boscardin, and A. K. Smith, "Lengths of Stay for Older Adults Residing in Nursing Homes at the End of Life," *Journal of the American Geriatric Society,* September 2010, Vol. 58.

4.14 Research, presentations, and publications at National Research Corporation, Lincoln, NE (internal and published).

4.15   Louise B. Andrew, M.D., J.D., "Physician Suicide: Overview" (Chief Editor: Barry E Brenner, M.D., Ph.D., FACEP), Medscape (Web page, updated June 1, 2016), http://emedicine.medscape.com/article/806779-overview.

4.16   American Foundation for Suicide Prevention, "Physician and Medical Student Depression and Suicide Prevention," (Web page, accessed February 22, 2016), http://afsp.org/our-work/education/physician-medical-student-depressionsuicide-prevention/.

4.17   M. N. Miller, K. Ramsey Mcgowen, and J. H. Quillen, "The Painful Truth: Physicians Are Not Invincible," *Southern Medical Journal*, 2000, 93(10).

4.18   USMLE Forum, "Re-entry to physician workforce problematic," (Web page blog entry, November 21, 2008), www.usmleforum.com/files/forum/2008/4/362392.php.

4.19   P. Wible, M.D., "Why Physicians Commit Suicide" (blog entry), December 12, 2012, www.idealmedicalcare.org/blog/why-physicians-commit-suicide/.

5.01   L. Leape, "Error in medicine," *Journal of the American Medical Association*, December 21, 1994, (272)23: 1851-1857.

5.02   V. Tellis-Nayak, "Who Will Care for the Caregivers?" *Health Progress*, November-December 2005, 866:37-43.

5.03   V. Tellis-Nayak, "The Satisfied but Disenchanted Leaders in Long-Term Care: The Paradox of the Nursing Home Administrator," *Seniors Housing & Care Journal*, 2007, 15:3-18.

5.04 National Center for Complementary and Integrative Health, "The Use of Complementary and Alternative Medicine in the United States: Cost Data," 2007 National Health Interview Survey, https://nccih.nih.gov/news/camstats/costs/costdatafs.htm.

5.05 M. Andrews, "Hospitals Offering Complementary Medical Therapies," *Kaiser Health News*, November 15, 2011 (citing a survey by the American Hospital Association and the Samueli Institute).

5.06 H. G. Koenig, M.D. "Religion, Spirituality, and Health: The Research and Clinical Implications," *ISRN Psychiatry*, 2012.

5.07 Pew Research Center, "America's Changing Religious Landscape," Demographic Study, May 12,2015, www.pewforum.org/2015/05/12/americas-changing -religious-landscape/.

5.08 C. M. Puchalski, "The Role of Spirituality in Health Care," Baylor University Medical Center Proceedings, October 2001, 14(4): 352–357.

5.09 V. Tellis-Nayak and M. Tellis-Nayak, "Games That Profesionals Play: The Social Psychology of Physician-Nurse Interaction," Social Science and Medicine, 1984, 18(12):1063-1069.

5.10 C. M. Puchalski, "The Role of Spirituality in Health Care," Baylor University Medical Center Proceedings, October 2001, 14(4): 352–357.

5.11 H. K. Silver, M.D. and A. D. Glicken, M.S.W., "Medical Student Abuse: Incidence, Severity, and Significance," *Journal of the American Medical Association,* January 26, 1990, 263(4): 527–532.

5.12 P. W. Chen, "The Bullying Culture of Medical School," The New York Times, August 9, 2011.

5.13   Editorial, "To Bully and Be Bullied: Harassment and Mistreatment in Medical Education," *AMA Journal of Ethics* (formerly *Virtual Mentor*), March 2014, 16(3): 155–160.

5.14   J. M. Fried, M. Vermillion, N. H. Parke, and S. Uijtdehage, "Eradicating Medical Student Mistreatment: A Longitudinal Study of One Institution's Efforts," *Academic Medicine*, September 2012, 87(9): 1191-1198.

5.15   L. Lenz, "Disruptive Behavior in Healthcare: Implications for Patients," Senior Seminar, University of Wisconsin, College of Education, 2008.

5.16   American College of Physician Executives, *Special Report: 2009 Doctor-Nurse Behavior Survey.*

5.17   *Ibid.*

5.18   T. Brown, RN, "Physician, Heel Thyself," *The New York Times* (op-ed), May 7, 2011.

5.19   S. J. Behrens, Letter to the Editor in response to T. Brown op-ed, *The New York Times*, May 8, 2011.

5.20   L. L. Leape, M. F. Shore, J. L. Dienstag, R. J. Mayer, S. Edgman-Levitan, G. S, Meyer, and G. B. Healy, "Perspective: A Culture of Respect, Part 1: The Nature and Causes of Disrespectful Behavior by Physicians," *Academic Medicine*, July 2012, 87(7): 845-85

5.21   E. Friedson, *Professional Dominance: The Social Structure of Medical Care*, Aldine Transaction Publishers, December 31, 2006.

5.22   American Board of Medical Specialties, 353 North Clark Street, Suite 1400, Chicago, IL, 60654.

5.23   Accreditation Board for Specialty Nursing Certification, www.nursingcertification.org.

5.24   D. Loxton, "The American Medical Association and the Fight Against Quackery," Insight at Skeptic.com (blog), June 14, 2015, www.skeptic.com/insight/the-american-medical-association-and-the-fight-against-quackery/.

5.25   B. Sabo, Ph.D., RN, "Reflecting on the Concept of Compassion Fatigue," *The Online Journal of Issues in Nursing*, 16(1), January 2011.

5.26   A. Verghese, M.D., "A Touch of Sense," *Health Affairs*, July/August 2009, 28(4): 1177–1182.

5.27   D. Keltner, "Hands On Research: The Science of Touch," The Greater Good Science Center, University of California at Berkeley, September 29, 2010, http://greatergood.berkeley.edu/article/item/hands_on_research.

5.28   C. Crist, "U.S. faces shortage of primary care doctors," *Georgia Health News*, October 5, 2013.

5.29   S. Thomson, R. Osborn, D. Squires, and M. Jun (editors), International Profiles of Health Care Systems, 2013, The Commonwealth Fund, November 2013.

5.30   The Physicians Foundation, *A Survey of America's Physicians: Practice Patterns and Perspectives* (survey conducted by Merritt Hawkins), September 2014.

5.31   L. Shi, "The Impact of Primary Care: A Focused Review," *Scientifica*, 2012.

5.32   P. J. Moore, N. E. Adler, and P. A. Robertson, "The effect of doctor-patient relations on medical patient perceptions and malpractice intentions," *Western Journal of Medicine*, October 2000, 1734: 244–250.

5.33   H. B. Beckman, K. M. Markakis, A. L. Suchman, and R. M. Frankel, "The Doctor-Patient Relationship and Malpractice: Lessons from Plaintiff Depositions," *Archives of Internal Medicine,* June 27, 1994, 154(12): 1365-1370.

5.34   The White House, Offices of the Press Secretary, "Clinton-Gore Administration Announces New Actions to Improve Patient Safety and Assure Health Care Quality," Press Release, February 22, 2000.

5.35   Institute for Healthcare Communication, "Impact of Communication in Healthcare," (Web page, accessed February 23, 2016), http://healthcarecomm.org/about-us/impact-of-communication-in-healthcare/.

5.36   M. Crane, "Wrong-Site Surgery Occurs 40 Times a Week," *Medscape Medical News,* June 29, 2011.

5.37   D. F. Mulloy and R. G. Hughes, "Chapter 36: Wrong-Site Surgery: A Preventable Medical Error," *Patient Safety and Quality: An Evidence-Based Handbook for Nurses* (R. G. Hughes, editor), Agency for Healthcare Research and Quality, April 2008.

6.01   E. O'Carroll, "Spain to Grant Some Human Rights to Apes," *The Christian Science Monitor,* June 27, 2008.

6.02   E. M. W. Tillyard and A. O. Lovejoy, "The Chain of Being: Tillyard in a Nutshell," (Web page, accessed June 10, 2016), https://web.cn.edu/kwheeler/Tillyard01.html.

6.03   S. Mcintyre, "Animals Are Now Legally Recognized as 'Sentient' Beings in New Zealand," *The Independent,* May 17, 2015.

6.04   "New EU Rules on Animal Testing Ban Use of Apes," *The Independent,* September 12, 2010.

6.05   B. Russell, *The Russell-Einstein Manifesto,* 1955.

6.06   A. H. Maslow, "A Theory of Human Motivation," *Psychological Review*, 1943, 50(4): 370-396.

6.07   H. Villarica, "Maslow 2.0: A New and Improved Recipe for Happiness," *The Atlantic*, August 17, 2011.

6.08   M. A. Max-Neef, *Human Scale Development: Conception, Application and Further Reflections*, Apex Press, December 1989.

6.09   A. Sen, *Development as Freedom*, Anchor (reprint edition), 2000.

6.10   M. Nussbaum, *Women and Human Development: The Capabilities Approach,* Cambridge University Press, June 2001.

6.11   Institute of Medicine, *To Err Is Human: Building a Safer Health System*, The National Academies Press, 1999.

6.12   Institute of Medicine, *Crossing the Quality Chasm: A New Health System for the 21st Century*, The National Academies Press, 2001.

6.13   National Research Corporation/Picker Institute, "Eight Dimensions of Patient-Centered Care," (Web page, accessed February 23, 2016), http://www.nationalresearch.com/products-and-solutions/patient-and-family-experience/eight-dimensions-of-patient-centered-care; and M. Gerteis, S. Edgman-Levitan, J. Daley, and T. L. Delbanco (editors), *Through the Patient's Eyes: Understanding and Promoting Patient-Centered Care*, Jossey-Bass, 1993.

6.14   *Ibid.*

6.15   See www.planetree.org; and www.pioneernetwork.net.

6.16   See www.pioneernetwork.net.

6.17   See www.edenalt.org.

6.18   See www.thegreenhouseproject.org.

7.01   R. Dawkins, *An Appetite for Wonder: The Making of a Scientist*, Harper Collins, 2013.

7.02   United States Conference of Catholic Bishops (USCCB), *A Culture of Life and the Penalty of Death: A Statement of the United States Conference of Catholic Bishops Calling for an End to the Use of the Death Penalty*, approved by the full body of bishops at the USCCB November 2005 General Meeting.

7.03   Universal Declaration of Human Rights, adopted by the United Nations General Assembly on December 10, 1948.

7.04   Kimberly Leonard, "Hospital of Yesterday: The Biggest Changes in Health Care," *U.S. News & World Report,* July 15, 2014.

7.05   "Healthcare of Tomorrow," *U.S. News & World Report* (Web page, accessed June 13, 2016), http://health.usnews.com/health-news/hospital-of-tomorrow?int=a2a909.

7.06   Institute of Medicine, *To Err Is Human: Building a Safer Health System*, The National Academies Press, 1999.

7.07   The Patient Safety and Quality Improvement Act of 2005 (PSQIA), Public Law 109-41, signed into law on July 29, 2005.

7.08   The Joint Commission, *What Did the Doctor Say? Improving Health Literacy to Protect Patient Safety*, 2007.

7.09   S. Harden, "Debriefing Improves Patient Safety," Safer Patients blog, July 9, 2015, http://saferpatients.com/blog/?p=69.

7.10   K. E. Schleiter, "Proving Causation in Environmental Litigation," *Virtual Mentor,* 2009, 11(6):456-460.

7.11   A. March, M.B.A., Ph.D. for the Health Research & Educational Trust (HRET), *Stories of Success: Using CUSP to Improve Safety,* Agency for Healthcare Research and Quality, 2012.

7.12   K. Curtiss, *Safe & Sound in the Hospital: Must-Have Checklists and Tools for Your Loved One's Care* (2nd Edition), PartnerHealth, LLC, 2012.

7.13   The Empowered Patient Coalition, http://empoweredpatientcoalition.org.

7.14   A. March, M.B.A., Ph.D. for the Health Research & Educational Trust (HRET), "What Is CUSP?" in *Stories of Success: Using CUSP to Improve Safety,* Agency for Healthcare Research and Quality, 2012.

7.15   Centers for Disease Control and Prevention, "Bloodstream Infection Event (Central Line-Associated Bloodstream Infection and Non-Central Line-Associated Bloodstream Infection), January 2016.

7.16   U.S. Department of Health & Human Services, "New HHS Data Shows Major Strides Made in Patient Safety, Leading to Improved Care and Savings," May 7, 2014.

7.17   K. Hobson, "Hospitals Make Progress on the Path to Safety," *U.S. News & World Report,* Aug. 13, 2014.

7.18   Patient Safety Network, "Getting Closer to the Bull's Eye: 2014–2015 Targeted Medication Safety Best Practices," *ISMP Medication Safety Alert! Acute Care Edition,* Agency for Healthcare Research and Quality, February 12, 2015; 20:1-5.

7.19   O. D. Guillamondegui, O. L. Gunter, L. Hines, B. J. Martin, W. Gibson, P. C. Clarke, W. T. Cecil, and J. B. Cofer, "Using the National Surgical Quality Improvement Program and the Tennessee Surgical Quality Collaborative to Improve Surgical Outcomes," *Journal of the American college of Surgeons,* Jan. 23, 2012; 214(4): 709-714.

7.20   Castlight Health, *Hand-Hygiene Safe Practices,* based on the 2014 Leapfrog Hospital Survey Results, The Leapfrog Group, 2014.

7.21   Patient Safety Network, "Getting Closer to the Bull's Eye: 2014–2015 Targeted Medication Safety Best Practices," *ISMP Medication Safety Alert! Acute Care Edition,* Agency for Healthcare Research and Quality, February 12, 2015; 20:1-5.

7.22   World Health Organization, "Road Traffic Injuries" (Web page, updated May 2016), http://www.who.int/mediacentre/factsheets/fs358/en/.

7.23   Capt. A. H. Wagner (Ret.) and Lt. Col. L. E. Baxton (Ret.), *Birth of A Legend: The Bomber Mafia and the Y1b-17,* Trafford Publishing, January 26, 2012.

7.24   Aircraft Owners and Pilots Association (AOPA), "General Aviation Safety Record - Current and Historic" (current as of March 2011; Web page, accessed June 10, 2016), www.aopa.org/about/general-aviation-statistics/general-aviation-safety-record-current-and-historic.

7.25   Anxieties.com, "How safe is commercial flight?" (Web page, accessed June 10, 2016), www.anxieties.com/flying-howsafe.php

7.26 Aircraft Owners and Pilots Association (AOPA), "General Aviation Safety Record - Current and Historic" (current as of March 2011; Web page, accessed June 10, 2016), www.aopa.org/about/general-aviation-statistics/general-aviation-safety-record-current-and-historic.

7.27 *Ibid.*

7.28 K. Hobson, "Hospitals Make Progress on the Path to Safety," *U.S. News & World Report,* Aug. 13, 2014.

7.29 É. Durkheim, *The Rules of Sociological Method*, originally published in 1895, translated by W. D. Halls, Free Press, December 1, 1982.

7.30 The W. Edwards Deming Institute, "The Theories and Teachings Are Nothing Short of Transformational in Spirit and in Practice," and "The Fourteen Points for Management," The Deming Institute, https://deming.org/theman/theories/fourteenpoints.

7.31 Suzanne Gordon, Patrick Mendenhall, Bonnie Blair O'Connor, *Beyond the Checklist: What Else Health Care Can Learn from Aviation Teamwork and Safety*, ILR Press, 2012.

7.32 A. Gawande, *The Checklist Manifesto,* Henry Holt and Company, 2009.

7.33 A. B. Haynes, M.D., M.P.H. et al., "A Surgical Safety Checklist to Reduce Morbidity and Mortality in a Global Population," *The New England Journal of Medicine,* Jan. 29, 2009; 360: 491-499.

7.34 A. Khoshbin, M.S.C., L. Lingard, Ph.D., and J. G. Wright, M.D., M.P.H., "Evaluation of Preoperative and Perioperative Operating Room Briefings at the Hospital for Sick Children," *Canadian Journal of Surgery*, August 2009; 52(4): 309-315.

7.35   S. Reinberg, "Safety Checklists for Surgery May Not Lower Deaths, Complications: Study," *HealthDay*, March 12, 2014.

7.36   A. Gawande, *The Checklist Manifesto,* Henry Holt and Company, 2009.

7.37   L. Lingard, S. Espin, S. Whyte, G. Regehr, G. Baker, R. Reznick, J.Bohnen, B. Orser, D. Doran, and E. Grober, "Communication Failures in the Operating Room: An Observational Classification of Recurrent Types and Effects," *Quality and Safety in Health Care,* Oct. 2004;13(5):330-334.

7.38   K. E. Schleiter, J.D., "Difficult Patient-Physician Relationships and the Risk of Medical Malpractice Litigation," *AMA Journal of Ethics,* March 2009, 11(3): 242–246.

7.39   A. Mozes, "Nursing Home Workers at Risk for Assault: Study," *HealthDay,* September 28, 2010.

7.40   My InnerView, *Annual National Report Staffing DMOG,* National Research Corporation, 2012.

8.01   N. S. Reiss and C. L. Tishler, "Suicidality in Nursing Home Residents: Part I and II," *Professional Psychology Research and American Foundation for Suicide Prevention,* Jun 2008; 39(3): 264-275.

8.02   "It Takes a Community," *Report on the Summit on Opportunities for Mental Health Promotion and Suicide Prevention in Senior Living Communities*, Gaithersburg, MD, October 16–17, 2008.

8.03   B. Mezuk, Ph.D., M. Lohman, Ph.D., M. Leslie, M.S., and V. Powell, Ph.D., "Suicide Risk in Nursing Homes and Assisted Living Facilities: 2003–2011," *American Journal of Public Health,* July 2015, 105(7): 1495-1502.

8.04   V. Tellis-Nayak and D. Ferguson, "The Social Construction of the Nursing Home: How Customers Interpret Nursing Home Life," *Seniors Housing & Care Journal,* 2013, 21(1): 86-99.

8.05   C. Rosen, J. Case, and M. Staubus, "Every Employee an Owner. Really.," *Harvard Business Review,* June 2005.

8.06   D. Weil, *The Fissured Workplace: Why Work Became So Bad for So Many and What Can Be Done to Improve It,* Harvard University Press, 2015.

8.07   B. Chewning, et al., "Patient Preferences for Shared Decisions: A Systematic Review," *Patient Education and Counseling,* January 2012, 86(1): 9–18.

8.08   A. Björnberg, "Patient Empowerment in Seven Key Countries," *Health Consumer Powerhouse,* March 13, 2013.

8.09   National Health Service, United Kingdom, Change 4 Life campaign, January 2009.

9.01   É. Durkheim, *Suicide: A Study in Sociology,* Free Press, 1951.

9.02   L. F. Berkman and L. Breslow, Health and Ways of Living: The Alameda County Study, Oxford University Press, 1983.

9.03   R. G. Rogers, R. A. Hummer, and C. B. Nam, Living and Dying in the USA: Behavioral, Health, and Social Differentials of Adult Mortality, Academic Press, 1999.

9.04   D. Umberson and J. K. Montez, "Social Relationships and Health: A Flashpoint for Health Policy," *Journal of Health and Social Behavior,* August 4, 2011, 51(Suppl.): S54-S66.

9.05 H. Liu and L. Waite, "Bad Marriage, Broken Heart? Age and Cardiovascular Risks Among Older Adults," *Journal of Health and Social Behavior,* December 2014, 55(4): 403–423.

9.06 L. J. Waite, E. O. Laumann, A. Das, and L. P. Schumm, "Sexuality: Measures of Partnerships, Practices, Attitudes, and Problems in the National Social Life, Health, and Aging Study," *The Journals of Gerontology, Series B: Psychological Sciences and Social Behavior,* Nov. 2009; 64(Suppl 1): i56-66.

9.07 J. T. Denney, B. K. Gorman, and C. B. Barrera, "Families, Resources, and Adult Health: Where Do Sexual Minorities Fit?" *Journal of Health and Social Behavior,* March 2013, 54(1): 46–63.

9.08 R. W. Simon, "Revisiting the Relationships among Gender, Marital Status, and Mental Health," *American Journal of Sociology,* January 2002, 107(4):1065-1096.

9.09 M. E. Hughes and L. J. Waite, "Marital Biography and Health at Mid-Life," *Journal of Health and Social Behavior,* September 2009, 50(3): 344–358.

9.10 L. J. Waite, "5 Marriage Myths, 6 Marriage Benefits," http://strongermarriage.org/divorce-remarriage/5-marriage-myths-6-marriage-benefits.

9.11 *Ibid.*

9.12 L. J. Waite and E. L. Lehrer, "The Benefits from Marriage and Religion in the United States: A Comparative Analysis," *Population and Development Review,* June 2003, 29(2): 255–276.

9.13   J. Levin, "Investigating the Epidemiologic Effects of Religious Experience," in J. Levin (editor), *Religion in Aging and Health: Theoretical Foundations and Methodological Frontiers,* SAGE Publications, Inc., October 20, 1993.

9.14   M. W. Frame, "The Spiritual Genogram in Family Therapy," *Journal of Marital and Family Therapy,* April 2000, 26(2): 211–216.

9.15   L. J. Waite, E. O. Laumann, A. Das, and L. P. Schumm, "Sexuality: Measures of Partnerships, Practices, Attitudes, and Problems in the National Social Life, Health, and Aging Study," *The Journals of Gerontology, Series B: Psychological Sciences and Social Behavior,* Nov. 2009; 64(Suppl 1): i56-66.

9.16   L. J. Waite, "The Negative Effects of Cohabitation," *The Communitarian Network,* Winter 1999/2000, 10(1).

9.17   L. J. Waite and E. L. Lehrer, "The Benefits from Marriage and Religion in the United States: A Comparative Analysis," *Population and Development Review,* June 2003, 29(2): 255–276.

9.18   H. G. Koenig, M.D., "Research on Religion, Spirituality, and Mental Health: A Review," *Canadian Journal of Psychiatry,* May 2009, 54(5): 283-291.

9.19   V. Tellis-Nayak, "The Transcendent Standard: The Religious Ethos of the Rural Elderly," *The Gerontologist,* 1982, 22(4): 359–363.

9.20   R. Schulz, Ph.D. and P. R. Sherwood, Ph.D., RN, CNRN, "Physical and Mental Health Effects of Family Caregiving," *American Journal of Nursing,* September 2008, 108(9 Suppl): 23–27.

9.21   C. G. Ellison and L. K. George, "Religious Involvement, Social Ties, and Social Support in a Southeastern Community," *Journal for the Scientific Study of Religion*, March 1994, 33(1): 46–61.

9.22   B. C. Booske, J. K. Athens, D. A. Kindig, H. Park, and P. L. Remington, *Different Perspectives for Assigning Weights to Determinants of Health*, County Health Rankings Working Paper, Population Health Institute, University of Wisconsin, February 2010.

9.23   J. R. Doty, M.D., "The Science of Compassion," *Huffpost Science*, The Huffington Post, June 7, 2012.

9.24   V. Tellis-Nayak, "The Satisfied but Disenchanted Leaders in Long-Term Care: The Paradox of the Nursing Home Administrator," *Seniors Housing & Care Journal*, 2007, 15: 3-18.

9.25   *Ibid.*

9.26   B. Lown, M.D., *The Lost Art of Healing: Practicing Compassion in Medicine*, Ballantine Books, February 1999.

9.27   D. Ofri, M.D., *What Doctors Feel: How Emotions Affect the Practice of Medicine*, Beacon Press, May 2014.

9.28   S. G. Post, Ph.D., "Compassionate Care Enhancement: Benefits and Outcomes," *The International Journal of Person Centered Medicine*, 1(4): 808–813.

9.29   F. S. Resnic, S. L. Normand, T. C. Piemonte, S. J. Shubroks, K. Zelevinsky, A. Lovet, and K. K. Ho, "Improvement in mortality risk prediction after percutaneous coronary intervention through the addition of a 'compassionate use' variable to the National Cardiovascular Data Registry CathPCI dataset: a study from the Massachusetts Angioplasty Registry," *Journal of the American College of Cardiology,* Feb. 22, 2011; 57(8): 904-911.

9.30   D. C. Dugdale, M.D., R. Epstein, M.D., and S. Z. Pantilat, M.D., "Time and the Patient–Physician Relationship," *Journal of General Internal Medicine,* January 1999; 14(Suppl 1): S34–S40.

9.31   D. R. Rhoades, K. F. McFarland, W. H. Finch, and A. O. Johnson, "Speaking and interruptions during primary care office visits," *Family Medicine,* July-August 2001, 33(7): 528-532.

9.32   K. E. Fletcher, G. Sharma, D. Zhang, Y. F. Kuo, J. S. Goodwin, "Trends in Inpatient Continuity of Care for a Cohort of Medicare Patients 1996-2006," *Journal of Hospital Medicine,* Oct. 2011; 6(8): 438-444.

9.33   J. D. Piette, Ph.D., M. Heisler, M.D., and T. H. Wagner, Ph.D., "Cost-Related Medication Underuse Among Chronically Ill Adults: The Treatments People Forgo, How Often, and Who Is at Risk," *American Journal of Public Health*, October 2004, 94(10): 1782–1787.

9.34   D. C. Dugdale, M.D., R. Epstein, M.D., and S. Z. Pantilat, M.D., "Time and the Patient–Physician Relationship," *Journal of General Internal Medicine,* January 1999, 14(Suppl 1): S34–S40.

9.35   D. Roter, "The Patient-Physician Relationship and its Implications for Malpractice Litigation," *Journal of Health Care Law and Policy,* 2006, 9(2): 304-314.

9.36   Institute for Healthcare Communication, "Team and Patient-Centered Communication Workshop," July 1 2011, http://healthcarecomm.org/2011/07/01/team-and-patient-centered-communication-work-shop/.

9.37   P. J. Moore, N. E. Adler, and P. A. Robertson, "Medical Malpractice: The Effect of Doctor-Patient Relations on Medical Patient Perceptions and Malpractice Intentions," *Western Journal of Medicine,* October 2000, 173(4): 244-250.

9.38   K. Kristof, "$1 Million Mistake: Becoming a Doctor," CBS MoneyWatch, September 10, 2013; and M. K. Nock, G. Borges, E. J. Bromet, C. B. Cha, R. C. Kessler.

9.39   A. Verghese, M.D., "The Way We Live Now: 3-16-03; Hard Cures," *The New York Times*, March 16, 2003.

9.40   J. Cassity, "The Science of Giving: Why One Act of Kindness is Usually Followed by Another," Happify Daily (Web page), www.happify.com/hd/the-power-of-a-single-act-of-kindness/.

9.41   D. McClelland and C. Kirshnnit, "The Effect of Motivational Arousal through Films on Salivary Immunoglobulin A," *Psychology & Health,* Dec. 19, 2007; pp. 31-52.

9.42   H. Stone, Ph.D., "Illness as Teacher," *Voice Dialogue International,* 2005.

10.01   V. J. Strecher, *On Purpose: Lessons in Life and Health from the Frog, The Dung Beetle, and Julia*, Dung Beetle Press, 2013.

10.02 A. H. Maslow, "A Theory of Human Motivation," *Psychological Review*, 1943, 50(4): 370-396.

10.03 Young@Heart Chorus, "20 Months of Making Music in Local Prisons," (Web page, accessed June 13, 2016), http://www.youngatheartchorus.com.

10.04 D. E. Yeatts, Ph.D., and C. M. Cready, Ph.D., "Consequences of Empowered CNA Teams in Nursing Home Settings: A Longitudinal Assessment," *The Gerontologist*, Jan. 8, 2007; 47(3): 323-339.

10.05 V. E. Frankl, *Man's Search For Meaning*, Beacon Press, 2006.

10.06 L. LaRose, "Purpose, Meaning, and Mental Health," Theravive, Nov. 12, 2014.

10.07 C. Weller, "Preserve Heart Health by Having a Purpose in Life," *Medical Daily*, Mar 6, 2015, www.medicaldaily.com/preserve-heart-health-having-purpose-life-324758.

10.08 V. E. Frankl, *Man's Search For Meaning*, Beacon Press, 2006.

10.09 H. Stone, Ph.D., "Illness as Teacher," *Voice Dialogue International*, 2005.

10.10 Gregory Orr, "Illness as Teacher," Barefoot and Laughing (blog), June 10, 2010.

10.11 P. Span, "Where the Oldest Die Now," *The New York Times*, April 18, 2012.

10.12 S. R. Kaufman, *And a Time to Die: How American Hospitals Shape the End of Life*, University of Chicago Press, 2006.

10.13 T. Brown, RN, "When It's the Doctor Who Can't Let Go," *The New York Times*, September 6, 2014.

10.14   A, Cirillo, "Dying with dignity: Lessons hospitals can learn from hospice," *Hospital Impact*, September 10, 2014.

10.15   P. Gozalo, Ph.D., J. M. Teno, M.D., S. L. Mitchell, M.D., M.P.H., J. Skinner, Ph.D., J. Bynum, M.D., M.P.H., D. Tyler, Ph.D., and V. Mor, Ph.D., "End-of-Life Transitions among Nursing Home Residents with Cognitive Issues," *The New England Journal of Medicine*, Sept. 29, 2011; 365: 1212-1221.

10.16   Avila Institute of Gerontology, Inc., Education for Compassionate Care, 600 Woods Rd., Germantown, NY 12526.

11.01   D. Keltner, *Born to Be Good: The Science of a Meaningful Life*, W. W. Norton & Company, October 5, 2009.

11.02   "Want to be happy? Giving is more gratifying than receiving," PBS News Hour, Jan 7, 2016, www.pbs.org/newshour/bb/want-to-be-happy-giving-is-more-gratifying-than-receiving/.

11.03   In-house research conducted by My InnerView, National Research Corporation.

11.04   V. E. Frankl, *Man's Search For Meaning*, Beacon Press, 2006.

11.05   M. Brock, A. Lange, and K. L. Leonard, "Generosity Norms and Intrinsic Motivation in Health Care Provision: Evidence from the Laboratory and the Field," European Bank for Reconstruction and Development, Working Paper No. 147, Aug. 2012.

11.06   G. Anand, "The Henry Ford of Heart Surgery - In India, a Factory Model for Hospitals Is Cutting Costs and Yielding Profits," *The Wall Street Journal*, Nov. 25, 2009.

Index

INDEX

About the Authors

The authors, a husband and wife team, have toiled in health care for a cumulative eighty-plus years. Individually or as a duo, they have conducted research and made presentations to academic and professional audiences across the fifty states in the United States and in several countries abroad. They have authored articles published in professional journals and trade magazines nationally and internationally; they have written standards, protocols, and survey instruments widely used by accrediting bodies and in business. In 2013, the American Health Care Association honored them with the Mary Ousley Champion of Quality Award in recognition of their contributions to quality in the long-term and post-acute care community. They continue to work in the field at the National Research Corporation.

CPSIA information can be obtained
at www.ICGtesting.com
Printed in the USA
LVHW030326151019
634227LV00001B/105/P